Milepost 75

Aging and Exploring Life Trails with Wonder, Resilience, and Love

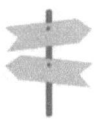

Sandra Richmond

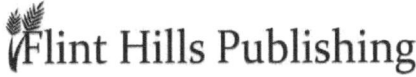
Flint Hills Publishing

PRAISE FOR MILEPOST 75

"Through generous vulnerability, wit, and wisdom, Sandra Richmond leads us to richer living, deeper intimacy, and enduring hope. More than a book, *Milepost 75* is loving mentoring in living well."

—Joseph Grenny
New York Times best-selling co-author of
Crucial Conversations and *Crucial Influence*

"This self-professed 'late bloomer,' took up an active lifestyle of walking/hiking in her 40s. Her memoir teaches us to dream big and then bigger, joyfully declaring that aging and life's journey do not have to be complicated if we take it one day at a time. If we put one foot in front of the other. If we trust the strangers, the 'angels' we meet on life's trails. If we trust ourselves to follow our dreams!"

—Sandra Kimberley Hall
15-year Himalayan trekker, award winning biographer/authority
of Hawaii's great Duke Paoa Kahanamoku

"Sandra Richmond is an engaging writer who has led a wonderfully active and aggressive life in 'old age'— something which I warmly endorse. If you're a serious hiker, this may be just the thing for you."

—Chris Crowley
New York Times best-selling co-author of *Younger Next Year*

.

"*Milepost 75* is part memoir, part travel guide, and part cheerleader. In it, Sandra Richmond talks about staying physically active as age overtakes us, but also about staying mentally and emotionally open to new experiences that age and wisdom provide. Sandra doesn't tell us what to do, or how to do it, but quietly encourages us to ask, 'Why not try it? It might be fun.'. It is at once a master class on aging and a celebration of a life fully lived."

—Melissa Bowersock
Award-winning author of multiple novels including
Ghost Walk and *Hopi Walk*

"You'll immediately connect with Sandra's heartfelt stories that inspire you to embrace life's many adventures. With vivid descriptions, she shares stories of cherished moments, strengthened relationships, and personal triumphs as well as failures. She steps outside her comfort zone, persists in the face of challenges, and savors the incredible rewards of pushing the limits to cross the finish line. She discovers the amazing rewards of doing JUST what she can, knowing it's exactly what she needs to do at the time. Whatever your age, prepare to be uplifted, inspired, and entertained as Sandra's powerful message empowers you to live life to the fullest, one step at a time."

—Lynn W. Murphy M.Ed.
Founder of Women Who Push the Limits, and author of
50 Life Lessons From Inspiring Women

"Sandra Richmond's inspirational book on her accomplishments and challenges of walking a multitude of varied trails in many countries, is filled with how she found joy, confidence, and friendships through perseverance, determination, and goals. She has a belief in herself and a passion for her sport that is equal to an elite athlete. She's proof that anyone at any level can be an athlete and how important it is to stay active as we age. Sandi is a wonderful example of how to face challenges and overcome them. Her experiences and inner drive can be applied to any goal one wants to achieve."

—Sarah Fredrickson
Competitive runner in elite competitions including the Ironman 140.6 Boulder and the Boston Marathon

---

"This inspiring book by Sandra Richmond shows how we don't need to be athletes to enjoy exercise, enjoy getting out in nature, and challenging ourselves. Although the author has had a number of medical challenges, she still walks every day around her neighborhood and regularly participates in longer events as well. Sandra truly has an indomitable spirit which drives her to set challenges for herself and rise to meet them no matter what her age."

—Hepsharat Amadi, M.D.

"This book is not a chronicle of hiking and competitive walking adventures, it is about taking responsibility for one's own health and wholeness, through hip and knee replacements, through the grief of life, to model physical and emotional health for self and others. Imagine (as I recommend), that you read this book every decade—in your 40s, 50s, 60s and on—as a chronicle of inspiration for your aging processes: to use this book as a guide for your determination to do your best to live well and change your yearnings into concrete and achievable goals. The best model for loving service to others is to healthfully love self and take responsibility for how you seek to be in the world. Sandra's soul says: "Don't just teach with words about hiking, walking, enduring—teach by being."

—Dr. Royce Fitts
Author of *The Geography of the Soul:*
Dreams, Reality, and the Journey of a Lifetime

Additional endorsements on the back cover from:

Jane Ramsey, author of *Vision Quest, a Journey to Happiness* and founder of Thriving in Retirement

Tom Zoellner, author of *Rim to River: Looking Into the Heart of Arizona*

Milepost 75
Aging and Exploring Life Trails
with Wonder, Resilience, and Love
© Sandra Richmond 2024
All rights reserved.

Map illustrations by Luisa Colón
www.luisacolon.com

Cover Design by Amy Albright
stonypointgraphics.weebly.com

Author photo by Melanie Miller

Flint Hills Publishing
Topeka, Kansas
Tucson, Arizona

www.flinthillspublishing.com

Printed in the U.S.A.

Paperback Book: ISBN 978-1-953583-74-1
Electronic Book ISBN 978-1-953583-76-5

Library of Congress Control Number 2023920682

Dedication

To Arnie, by my side,
making this journey possible,
filling it with joy.

Contents

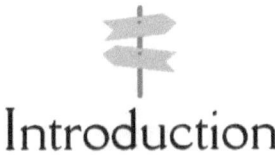

Introduction

"You can't keep walking so much!" Dr. Sofia Mendez exclaimed in frustration. "You'll wear out your implants." My sports medicine doctor stared at the X-ray of my artificial hips. She shook her head, turned, looked hard at me. "Sandi, you must find something else. Swimming and biking are fine but not all this walking."

"That's not an option," I blurted out. "Not now. Not for my quality of life!" *Whoa! Where did that come from*? I pride myself on being a good patient. I listen. I follow directions. But my passionate reaction emerged from my heart and flew out of my mouth before I really knew what happened. I think we were both surprised.

Dr. Mendez had treated me last year for bursitis pain in my left hip. I tend to avoid getting cortisone shots and had waited until this year's pain was affecting my critical daily activities. Now I could barely walk. The shooting pain was in my right hip this time. She didn't think it was aggravated by my joints at this point, but she could see the potential chaos of all the miles I was putting on my implants.

We sat still and silent in her office, each of us dealing with our own inner turmoil.

I looked down trying to get a grip. I was determined to keep walking, but she was scaring me. *What if I can't keep going? I know I'll eventually have to cut back on walking this much, but I have such super plans for my 75th year. There's no way I'm going to stop all my training walks. Not now. I need at least one more year.*

I bunched up my shoulders and bit my bottom lip. *Maybe she's right. But maybe not.*

I looked up. We locked eyes. We stared at each other for another awkward minute. I took a big breath and another. I knew she wanted what was best for me. She was genuinely concerned about my aging artificial apparatuses. She wanted me to be reasonable. I was in no mood. I sat still. Stared back.

When it became obvious I was not going to budge, Dr. Mendez sighed and said, "Okay. One more year, then we'll talk. But what else are you doing right now in addition to walking to stay strong and build muscle around your joints?"

Good question! I could show her I wasn't *totally* focused on walking for my fitness and well-being. "I take ballet exercise and Tai Chi classes twice a week, ride my stationary bike at home, and do strength, balance, and flexibility exercises 2-3 times a week."

She smiled. "Good! Keep that up, especially the ballet exercise. Work on strengthening your hip and leg muscles so they keep cushioning and supporting your joints."

She gave me the shot and a list of exercises to help alleviate the bursitis. I headed out of her office with renewed resolve. This was it. I had to treat next year as my best and maybe my last year of big events.

Dr. Mendez added a mega dose of reality. My artificial hips were almost fifteen years old with a life-expectancy of 20 years. My knees weren't too far behind. There was a strong possibility that they would wear out before I did.

Soon after my appointment, I created a 4x6 list of all the things I wanted to do next year. Most adventures, events, and activities were on my 2019 calendar, and I was already training for them. They included several half marathons, some 5Ks, the American Lung Association Fight for Air stair climb, a Sierra Club 50K One Day Hike and a Grand Canyon one-day rim-to-rim hike (R2R). I'd probably add a few more things. This would be my way to celebrate turning 75. All year long.

I felt a tiny tinge of trepidation regarding my arthritic feet. I'd worry about them later. Thank goodness I didn't mention them to Dr. Mendez!

People ask if I've always been an avid walker. The answer is no. I am a late starter, not even finding my true passion of hiking, walking, and climbing until I turned 45.

The first hike that ignited my passion was a Grand Canyon Rim-to-Rim-to-Rim (R2R2R). A 50-mile 24-hour hike that would probably be considered an *ultramarathon* today.

After my Grand Canyon awakening, I began to wonder if I could write a book. That notion meandered in my mind for years, along with the question: "Why would anyone be interested?"

I have big goals and tackle challenging adventures, but I'm not a natural-born athlete. I've never been a runner. Never been the best or fastest at anything. I'm generally healthy with no major physical issues to overcome. I'm a walker, a slow walker. There are many women my age who hike, run, and walk much faster than I do. My story is not about coming from behind and ending up in first place. I usually cross the finish line with a few others behind me. I've earned a few awards when I'm the oldest or only person in the age group. Then I win because I'm old, not fast.

I had six months, from June through December, to enhance my health, improve my stamina, and increase my strength. And then I decided to capture that other lurking objective. Write a book. Tell my story.

I'm willing to embrace tough adventures when I'm not at my best, even with the possibility that I may not be able to finish. I get scared when I consider doing something intimidating, but I don't let that fear prevent me from doing it. And so, although this was especially daunting, I decided now was the right time to capture this dream.

When I wonder if anyone would read this book, be inspired or motivated by it, I remember that woman in Portland, Maine.

I never had a Bucket List. The only time I played with the idea of *doing something before I die* was back in 2013 when my daughter, Rachel, and I were in Portland the day before the annual "Tri for a Cure" sprint triathlon, a 1/3-mile swim in the Atlantic, 15-mile bike ride, and a 5K run.

"C'mon, Mom," Rachel had said on the phone in January, just before I turned 69. "Let's both enter the lottery for this event. It's very popular and fills up quickly. If one of us gets selected, we can relay. I'll do the swim and run, and you can do the bike. It is *highly* unlikely we'll both get selected. Even if we don't get selected at all, we will have donated to a good cause. What do you say?"

I said yes.

We both got selected.

Of course.

We rented wet suits for the first time ever and trained for our Atlantic Ocean swim in pools and ponds. We were equally terrified. Both of us worried about me!

As usual, we turned this event into a family adventure, so my son-in-law, Rob, and teenage grandsons Andrew and Jonathan joined us. We had just finished eating our very first lobster rolls and were walking around the pier looking for an ice cream shop. We stopped in front of a rustic restaurant and studied a big blackboard standing on a wooden frame with the words: "The One Thing I Want to Do Before I Die, is…" The entire board was filled with handwritten dreams, wishes, and goals floating in waves of colored chalk—a beautiful piece of poetry in motion:

> Run a marathon.
> See a Broadway play. Complete an Ironman.
> Run a marathon. (*There were a lot of these*)
> Hike the Grand Canyon (*Been there, done that*).
> Hike the AT.
> Get kissed by Brad Pitt. (*…a lot of these too*)

"What's the one thing you want to do, Mom?" Rachel asked.

I hesitated, slowly picked up a piece of turquoise chalk, my favorite color, then took the plunge, "Write a book." I had journals scattered all over but had never gotten around to actually writing a book. So that became the solitary entry in my bucket.

Now it was official. I finally planted the seed that had been blowing in the wind for so many years.

And that seed was watered the next day when Rachel and I completed the sprint triathlon. I placed third, significantly behind the other two women in my 65-69 age group. My backstroke, sidestroke, flapping-flipping swim time was pathetic. I picked up a little time in biking. Then lost time again in the 5K when I headed out the wrong gate, got redirected, and walked out the right gate as fast as I could go.

After the ceremony, we gathered round to admire my 3rd place award—an adorable multi-color bejeweled silver-painted plastic tiara.

As we stepped aside, waiting for the crowds to thin out so we could pick up our bikes, a young woman walked up. She gently tapped me on the shoulder and said, "I just want you to know that I finished this event because of you."

"Me?" I blinked. Crooked my head.

"Yes. You. This was my first sprint triathlon. I had biked into transition depleted, discouraged, and done, totally ready to call it quits. Then I saw you, smiling, striding, slapping your cap on your shiny grey hair and heading out of the transition area way behind most others. I flung my bike on the rack, headed out on the 5K, looking, pacing myself with your white cap bobbing ahead. I walked and watched and repeated to myself, 'If she can keep going, so can I.' You crossed the finish line. And, because of you, so did I. Thank you."

I was slow, way behind most others. And yet I inspired her.

I'm writing this book for that woman.

I love seeing active women (and men) in their late seventies, eighties, even nineties. How do they get healthy and stay moving? How hard is it for them? What keeps them going? Where do they find their passion and perseverance? These elders encourage and inspire me to follow in their footsteps, to stay healthy and happily active. Perhaps the story of my 75th year will help do the same for others, especially those who find it frustrating, intimidating, and challenging to stay active as we age.

And there is no doubt I am aging. I'm often tempted to keep these issues to myself, carrying them around as extra baggage. But I push myself to be open with my doctors, my husband Arnie, and my good friends who are dealing with many of the same challenges. Sharing struggles with kindred souls helps me laugh, allows me to gain perspective.

Not only has my body changed, but also my spirit. After I retired and entered my 70s, I became more fearless. More curious. More willing to step way out of my comfort zone. More willing to embrace emerging exciting experiences. My world and life expanded. I started taking at least one challenging trip each year including a 4-day, 3-night Inca Trail Trek in Peru with my daughter, an 8.5 K fun run/walk on the Great Wall in China with my son and grandson, and a 50K Sierra Club One Day Hike along the C&O Canal with another grandson. Arnie stayed home, encouraging me to follow my dreams and cheering me in spirit all the way.

I knew I would travel more when I retired, but I *never* dreamed I would take things this far.

This book is *not* about giving advice. It *is* about how I dealt with challenges, opportunities, and roadblocks. Making mistakes. Usually finishing. Sometimes not. Learning lessons. Exploring options. Never giving up. It's written with humor (most of the time) and gratitude (all the time). Reporting, not complaining, because I'm incredibly thankful for my health and ability to stay active, to be fully alive and enjoy each day.

Sandra Richmond

I'll share love and gratitude for my beloved husband Arnie who encourages and supports me, and the rest of my family who are with me in some way on every trail.

And I will give thanks for my body that is growing older, getting stronger in some ways, breaking down in others, but still moving forward, one step at a time.

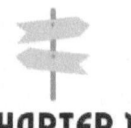

CHAPTER 1
Milepost 45:
Finding My Starting Line

HAVE YOU ALWAYS WANTED TO WRITE AN ARTICLE? PITCH IT? MAYBE EVEN GET IT PUBLISHED?"

That yellow flyer grabbed my attention with its bold, blaring headline. Posted on a bulletin board of the telephone company where I worked, it was almost buried in the ephemeral detritus of ads, announcements, updates, and reminders.

Easy for someone to miss. But not me.

The flyer announced a class held in a small office building on my way home from work, where we lived in Tucson, Arizona. The class met weekly and early enough that I could still get home for dinner with Arnie and the kids. How fortuitous! An opportunity to learn something new. Maybe this is what would help me get unstuck.

I signed up. Sat in the first session with seven other women. The goal of this class was for each of us to write at least one "publishable" article by the end of the six-week course. Nice!

Our instructor, Nancy, walked into the room. She was statuesque and trim, with auburn hair pulled back into a neat ponytail, wearing a white tailored blouse tucked neatly in belted brown trousers. Right on time. She smiled and introduced herself. Then asked us to go around the room doing the same, giving our names, explaining we would get to know more about each other through our class activities.

After introductions, Nancy gave us our first assignment: to sit quietly and think of one or two things we want help with. "If you have a question, there's a good chance others want to know the same thing, and it might make a great article," she explained. "The questions can be hard, easy, common, or unique. Okay? Ready to start? Any questions?" We chuckled. Nancy smiled, "Okay, get to work on your question for the group. Take your time. Relax and let your mind discover some things you'd really like to know."

We eight women leaned back in our chairs. I closed my eyes and opened my mind.

The big question floating around in my head regarded my ennui. I had been content for many years, working at the telephone company, living a good life, and feeling perfectly balanced. Why now did I feel dissatisfied and even guilty? So many people had much bigger struggles. Our children were healthy. We were doing reasonably well. Was this a mid-life crisis? And if so, what could I do about it?

At some point I had stopped breathing, then (wisely) decided to take a breath and get a grip. I settled down and tried to come up with a more appropriate, less existential question for this group.

I sat back. This time more curious, wistful, searching. *What question do I have for this group?* I thought. *What is something aspirational, even attainable?*

And it came to me. I love the Grand Canyon and want to see even more of it. A clear and straightforward question that had been lurking in the back of my mind for years popped into my brain. That was it! I had my question.

"Okay," Nancy asked. "Is everyone ready? Remember this is a judgement-free exercise. Who wants to go first?"

"I will," said a woman across the table from me. "I love houseplants. When I go into someone's house, it's the first thing I see and admire. But when I go shopping, I can't seem to find the right plants. And when I do and bring them home, they all die. Can any of you help me figure this out?"

I offered to go next. "Do any of you know of a way to hike across the Grand Canyon from the South Rim to the North Rim without backpacking, in a short period of time, and very cheap?"

There was dead silence. I looked around the table. Saw mostly glazed eyes and open jaws. *Thank goodness I didn't go with my first question!*

After what felt like three hours—but was really only a few more seconds—one woman asked, "Why would you want to do that?" Her tone was kind. It wasn't like she was sneering, "Why in the hell would you want to do that?" She sounded genuinely interested.

I ignored the gasps and raised eyebrows. "I'm not really sure myself," I said. "But I can't shake this dream. About five years ago, a friend invited me to hike to the bottom, camp one night, and then hike back out the next day. She was an experienced backpacker. I was not. She assured me I'd be fine."

That kind woman gave me an encouraging nod. "The first portion of the hike down South Kaibab Trail was steep and beautiful, other worldly, with so much green! But as we got closer to the bottom, the 107-degree heat became suffocating. Worst of all, my backpack felt like a block of concrete weighing me down and pushing out every ounce of joy from my body."

She kept gently probing, "Why would you want to do this if that first hike was so terrible?"

"The heat was oppressive, but the heavy backpack felt even more crushing," I explained. "The hike was beautiful. I just wanted to move unincumbered and soak it all in. Every switchback on this steep and rocky trail offered new views I had never seen before. The inner canyon is a magical place, and it's right in our back yard, sort of. It's just a six-hour drive from Tucson to the South Rim."

I described how we found our campsite in the Bright Angel campground and pitched our tent. We even quickly splashed in, dunked down, and rushed out of the freezing Bright Angel Creek. We got up at 3:00 the next morning, ate a quick breakfast, and were on the trail by 4:00 to climb up Bright Angel Trail, hiking in the dark as far as we could before the sun's rays started to beat on our bodies and blister the trail. We had flashlights. It was cool. We could manage the heat. I could not manage my frustration with lugging that heavy backpack.

"After hours and miles, now in the full sun, we rested in a shady spot along the trail. Just then, a guy sauntered up wearing a fanny pack. He *sauntered*! He walked straight. No slouch. No backpack. He told us he had hiked down to the bottom starting at midnight from South Kaibab trailhead to beat the heat and was hiking back up the Bright Angel Trail in the same day! He carried a light load with a flashlight, snacks, extra socks, and was able to refill his three water bottles along the way."

At this point, one woman started tapping her pen on the table; another cleared her throat. *I need to wrap this up.*

I paused. The room stayed quiet. Except for that tapping pen. (Getting louder)

"And that's what I want to do. I want to be that guy. I want to hike long and far, see as much of the canyon as possible, and do it without camping and carrying a heavy backpack."

"I have your answer!" another woman piped up.

The pen tapping stopped.

"My husband is a member of the Southern Arizona Hiking Club, and he knows someone named Sid Hirsh who leads *exactly* the kind of hike you're looking for. It's called a rim-to-rim-to-rim Grand Canyon hike. The goal is to hike from the South Rim to the North Rim and back to the South Rim all in one day. No camping. No heavy backpack. Just a flashlight and daypack for snacks and water."

That was it! All I had to do was call Sid and start training. I left that meeting with a new spring in my step, hope in my heart, and an answer to my second question.

But I still needed an answer to my first question, the one I didn't ask in the meeting: How can I pull myself back together and get unstuck, back to my feeling of balance and contentment?

Before I could even start to figure that out, a solution popped up in my email. "This is a voluntary offer to all managers who are at least 45 years old and have 20 years of service. The company will add five years to your service and five years to your age, making you eligible for full retirement. And as an added incentive you can receive your retirement as a one-time bonus and receive lifetime medical coverage."

I was 45. In January 1990 I would celebrate my 20th anniversary with the company. I could be eligible to "retire." This was the answer to my first question. Taking this offer would certainly get me unstuck.

But it couldn't. It was out of the question. The amount of the pension buyout was significant but earnings from that investment would amount to much less than my current salary. We hadn't saved enough to fill in the gap.

I listened to Paul, one of my peers, a trusted advisor. "You make a good salary. You'll never make this much money starting over at this point in your life." (Has-been at 45? Apparently so.)

My career at US West had been educational and satisfying mainly because my leader, Ruel Cooper, was willing to take a chance on me by placing me in non-traditional leadership positions. He was my first mentor, and he opened the biggest doors to my current and future leadership success. My skills were not typical, not technical. I had a BS in education, a Masters in counseling and guidance, and an affinity for bonding and building productive teams using strategic group results to track and celebrate.

Most recently, Ruel took a significant risk by placing me in an engineering manager role, even though I had no formal engineering training or background. This was new. It had never been done before. But Ruel saw my willingness to work hard, learn, and get results. It was the right time for more diversity. To test new waters. I had several mentors throughout my career, but Ruel was the first and he got me started on the right path.

This new engineering manager role was a challenge for me, but even more so for the longtime engineers who thrived and valued the status quo—the way things had always been done, the right way. My presence was threatening. Totally new. I became a student of my new team, meeting with each member of my staff, creating alignment and a collegial productive bond with most, but not all. Through this onboarding process, I learned valuable skills that helped me navigate new leadership positions throughout the rest of my career at US West and other organizations.

But even the most demanding stimulating roles can become routine. By now most of that groundbreaking, interesting work was done. And with this deep, steep downsizing, the company would be static, stabilizing for at least the next few years. I was already getting bored.

As Arnie and I cleaned up dinner that night, I off-handedly mentioned the offer, not even filling in all the details since it was out of the question. "Are you sure you don't want to consider this?" he asked. "It's risky, but I think we may both be ready for a change."

Arnie had become the stay at-home parent when Rachel was born in 1976 (back in the dark ages before flexible family lifestyles became popular) and continued to embrace that role when Jonathan was born four years later. Our decision worked well for us based on our inclinations and abilities. We were both raised by divorced working mothers, and were comfortable living in the margins of what was considered *normal*. No role models.

No social media. We figured things out on our own, what worked best for us and our growing family, charting our own path.

I was the main breadwinner, joyfully juggling work during the day and spending precious family time in the evenings and weekends. Taking walks. Reading books. Exploring museums. Being together.

Arnie was the homemaker, caretaker. He volunteered in their classrooms. Played games with them. Told stories.

Sometimes I even cooked. But I was impatient. (Still am.) I cooked everything on high and usually wandered away to do something else. (Still do.) In fact, several years later, the kids were stunned to learn that all scrambled eggs were *not* brown and tough, and all French Toast was *not* black and rock hard.

Our decision to switch roles had worked well for many years. But Arnie was right. Lately we both wanted more. He missed the challenge of a career outside the home.

I wanted more time at home with Arnie and the kids. More sweet moments with my elderly mom. More camping trips. Discovering a new world outside the structure of full-time work. I even resurrected a discarded dream of going back to the University of Arizona to earn a PhD—something I had wanted to do for years but was impossible to accomplish on a part-time basis.

But I continued to listen to my head and even told my boss: "I'm 100% sure I'm staying." Taking this offer was simply not realistic.

One evening as we strolled around the block hanging back behind the kids, Arnie persisted: "We will have more time and less money. We don't know how things will work out, but it's an opportunity to start over, to reinvent ourselves. Please consider this. We can do this together. We can make it work."

I started to listen. Started to consider. This offer would add five years to our age and our service and was quickly dubbed the 5+5. We 5+5 candidates attended a transition workshop and listened as the facilitator gave us our first assignment. "Describe your life five years from now in 1995." I quickly scribbled, "Rachel would be 19, Jonathan 15, Mom 80." I paused, then continued to write. "If I stay at work and maybe end up working even more hours in a downsized organization, I may miss out on major opportunities to spend time with Arnie, the kids, and my mom. To follow my dreams. So many life experiences are fleeting. So many things cannot be put on hold."

That night I told Arnie, "If I turn down this offer, stay at work, and then die in five years, I will *not* be amused. What good would all that security do us then?"

With two more weeks before the deadline I kept receiving *coaching*. One company leader called. "Sandi, I talked this over with one of the other VPs and here's what we think. Since you weren't at home with Rachel and Jonathan when they were little, you've already blown it. They've done all the cute stuff and want to spend time with their friends. You might as well stay at work."

Yet another leader up the chain of command called. "Sandi, you're making a big mistake. This is the time to stay, not leave. We need you and there will be so many more opportunities in a smaller, leaner company."

Arnie's message persisted. Slowly seeping into my head and shoving aside all those needs for status quo, security, and stability. Finally, I listened and decided to accept the offer.

So, at a time when many women were expanding their work roles, I chose to expand my mom role. When most people had completed their education many years earlier, I was considering going back to school to earn a doctorate. When most people our age were diligently saving for retirement, Arnie and I were going to spend this pension to shake up our lives and explore a new universe of opportunities.

We clasped our hands, took a deep breath, and jumped into uncharted waters. We knew we could flail but also thrive in turbulent waves. We promised we would be each other's life preservers. That we would never look back.

We never did.

A jigsaw puzzle of our life before this change would have had straight borders. A clear picture with large pieces that easily fit together. Our new puzzle would have a haphazard border with lots of pieces that may not fit neatly together. We had no idea how this new life panorama would turn out. But we started putting together our new puzzle of life. One piece at a time.

We quickly made changes. More camping trips. More relaxing dinners on the picnic table in our backyard. Always cooked by Arnie. Of course. Arnie went back to college, started a part-time job as executive director of our synagogue, and continued to coach Jonathan in little league. I secured a part-time job, teaching night classes for the University of Phoenix.

I took the GMAT PhD entrance exam after studying on my own. But my percentile was not high enough to get accepted. My brain had slowed over the years. I needed to work harder, get faster and better.

I could not start my PhD program that first year. But what I *could* do is call Sid Hirsh.

"Hi, Sid? My name is Sandi Richmond and I heard you lead a Grand Canyon hike called the rim-to-rim-to-rim. I was wondering if I could join you." I paused. Then added, "And maybe even my daughter, Rachel."

"Oh, absolutely!" Sid said in his bright tone. "And if Rachel comes, you two will be our first mother-daughter team! This event is really catching on. We just completed our hike for this year so you and your daughter will have an entire year to train for the next one in May of 1991. You should join the Southern Arizona Hiking Club if you're not a member. They go on hikes all the time. And even if you don't want to join them you can read the newsletter and learn about the best trails you and your daughter can hike on your own."

Sid was in a hurry, but he couldn't seem to stop himself. "Just so you know, this is more than *just* a rim-to-rim-to-rim hike. It's a special hike called the "Rim-to-Rim-to-Rim 50/24 (R2R2R-50/24) that we initiated a few years ago. Instead of hiking straight down Bright Angel to Phantom Ranch on the way down, we added a little connecting hike on the Tonto Trail over to the South Kaibab Trail. So now it's at least 50 miles instead of 47."

Sid finally took a breath. "That's probably enough information for now. I have to hang up and get going but go ahead and get started. We can talk later. Bye."

This was a big deal. I might not make it the first time. But the clock was ticking. I was hooked. So, I made a pledge to myself to complete the entire 50 miles in 24 hours by the time I turned 50. I believed in my heart of hearts that if I couldn't do it by then, I never would.

At this point, everything was coming together. I wasn't sure Rachel would be as excited about this opportunity as I was, especially since she had never hiked in the Grand Canyon before. But I thought it would be a sweet mother-daughter experience.

So, I asked her.

She said yes!

Rachel and I had started walking together when she was just eight years old. She was a natural athlete: strong, coordinated, tough. She did not care for team sports like her brother, but she was always delighted to go walking with me. We started walking around the block. Then I added more distance, different routes. When she would start to get bored, I'd toss some dimes ahead on the trail when she wasn't looking. "Rachel, look at the trail. There's something shiny."

Rachel would perk up. Lose her boredom. Get curious. Start searching the path. "Oh Mom, look! Another dime!" Finding coins on the path turned our walks into adventures. Sometimes she'd come home with almost a dollar.

Our walks grew longer. Both of us discovering new delights. Being outside. Being with nature. Being together in an entirely new way as partners. We walked and talked about movies and books. We chatted about the bushes, bugs, and birds we saw on our walks. We were also content walking in silence, just spending time outside together.

Our long-walk training had started a few years before the R2R2R-50/24 opportunity when I was chairperson of the local March of Dimes board. Their main fund raiser was the Super Walk: 30 kilometers around the Tucson city streets. After the first few years of walking with my friends, I asked Rachel and two of her friends to join us. By then she no longer needed coins to motivate her. We walked even more miles. Training together. Just for the fun of it.

Rachel was ready for something bigger. We immediately started training for next May's hike. I joined the Southern Arizona Hiking Club and read each newsletter. We trained on many of the same trails they hiked.

Most of our hikes were in the mountains, but we did city walks too. One Saturday, Arnie dropped us off at dawn on the west side of Tucson. We walked all the way to our home on the east side. More than 20 miles. October weather was mild. We stopped at convenience stores for drinks and restroom breaks. Ate lunch at Subway. And sat outside at a Dairy Queen savoring a well-deserved peanut buster parfait toward the end of our walk. I don't remember how long we walked or what we talked about, but I will always remember how good it felt.

We bought slightly bigger boots when we discovered our blisters usually started after 15 miles of hiking and our feet began to swell. We trained hard and completed multiple long, challenging hikes including two 25-milers on steep mountain trails in the Rincon mountain range by the time next April rolled around.

I called Sid again.

"Hi there!" he responded in the same excited tone. "I didn't see your name on any of the hike rosters, so I was wondering if you and your daughter were going to join us."

"The newsletter has been great," I responded. "But it was more convenient for us to go out on our own."

Silence. "Super! The point is you've been training. This time a journalist from *Arizona Highways* is joining us to write an article about the hike. Some of us will meet the night before for a spaghetti dinner, but most people will just join us at 3:00 a.m. at Bright Angel Lodge for the briefing before we head out."

"Thanks, Sid. We'll see you at the lodge in the morning."

"Great! We will have more than 60 hikers this year, a new record. And we'll probably have even more next year once that article gets published. Okay, see you Saturday morning. Gotta go."

Sid hung up.

We had three weeks before the hike. Ample time for me to panic. When I took Jonathan for his annual physical, I checked with our pediatrician: "Dr. Dew, Rachel and I are planning to hike the Grand Canyon rim-to-rim-to-rim in a few weeks and I'm starting to worry this will be too much for her."

He smiled and responded, "Some of my friends are members of the Southern Arizona Hiking Club and they did that big hike last year. Rachel is 15. She's young, healthy, and strong. She will be fine. But what about you? That's a pretty big thing to do for the first time at 47. You're the one who's taking a big step."

And before we knew it, it was showtime. Arnie sent us off with his usual high hopes and encouragement. "I know it will be impossible to call during the hike, but please keep me posted as much as you can. You will be fine. Be careful and have fun. Love you."

Early Friday the day before the hike, Rachel and I drove up to the Grand Canyon. We listened to country CDs. Rachel read the

People Extra Summer issue of "The 50 Most Beautiful People in The World 1991" with Julia Roberts on the cover.

We checked into Kaibab Lodge on the South Rim down the road from Bright Angel Lodge where we would join the group the next morning. We unpacked and walked down to Kaibab Lodge cafeteria for dinner on our own. Our stomachs churned. It was hard to eat our carb-packed spaghetti and meatball dinner. It was even challenging to eat more than a few bites of the tasty garlic toast.

We went back to our room and laid out all our stuff. We packed all the snacks that had worked well on our training hikes: PB&Js, pretzels, orange slices, bananas, peanut M&M's, Gatorade powder.

We went to bed around 8:00 p.m. Tossed and turned most of the night, thinking of the big unknown that tomorrow would bring. The alarm went off at 1:30 am.

"Did you sleep much?" I asked.

"I don't think so," Rachel responded.

"Me neither," I said. "We can snack on the trail, but I think we should try to eat something now."

"Mom, there is no way. Can we at least wait until just before we start?"

"Sure. I can't eat either."

We shivered as we headed out to the car in the misty air. "Mom! Look!" Rachel exclaimed. There was a deer standing there watching us, glowing under the aura of a lone streetlight. "For some reason, that makes me feel good," she said.

"Me too."

We drove to Bright Angel Lodge and walked up the front steps. Bright lights from big windows created an inviting glow and confirmation we were in the right place. I still said to myself: *I hope this is the right place.* Even though it was one of the few things I knew for sure.

We tugged open the door. A mighty noise embraced us and pulled us into a crowded cavernous room, packed with hikers of all shapes and sizes, dressed in varying assortments of clothes and trail paraphernalia hanging on their backs or around their hips. Everyone was chattering. Most folks seemed to know each other or were quickly introducing themselves. Rachel and I stood to the side to take it all in. We were overwhelmed.

Then I heard that voice. "Okay everybody! Gather round. It's time for last minute instructions."

Sid Hirsh stood on the hearth of the giant stone fireplace at the far end of the rustic hotel lobby. "I see a lot of new folks joining us. Welcome! Just a few things to remember. As you know, we'll head down Bright Angel Trail to Indian Garden. Then we'll take a sharp right turn onto Tonto Trail. Now this is the one spot that's easy to miss, although it should be daylight for most of you when you get here. And, when you return, you'll just come straight up Bright Angel Trail."

Rachel looked at me, eyes wide. A man noticed her concern. "He's talking about the Tonto Trailhead just beyond the pump station as you leave Indian Garden. Keep looking to the right and you'll see it. You'll be fine." He smiled. We smiled, feeling a bit better.

Sid continued. "Please let runners go first. Take care of yourself and be courteous to others so we all make it back here safely."

Rachel looked at me again, her eyes even bigger. "Some people are running this?" The kind man leaned in again. "Some folks will be running but most of us will be hiking steadily and carefully. Just let the runners go ahead and you'll be fine. You do not want to get in their way," he said, shaking his head.

"And finally," Sid continued, "as you all should know, while it's chilly on the rim, by the time you get to the bottom it will be like hiking in Tucson, probably hotter than 100 degrees. You will descend more than 4,300 feet in elevation during your first 12 miles or so."

Sid stopped. He waited for the ambient chatter to die down. "Please, please understand and remember the absolute hottest portion of this hike is the box. For those of you who don't know, this is a tight deep canyon along Bright Angel Creek shortly after you leave Phantom Ranch. Pace yourself and be safe but do your best to get through the box before the sun is directly overhead. Canyon walls are so steep and narrow in this section it can turn into a burning radiating oven."

Sid paused. Dead silence. Waiting for that warning to sink in. "Okay? Okay! That's it. Let's get going."

More than sixty people lined up. There was a stampede of early starters running to the trailhead. It was almost 4:00. A few hours before dawn. By the time Rachel and I and other hikers reached the trail we could already see flickering flashlights lighting up the switchbacks like a shiny ribbon of fireflies. We waited for a few more runners to rush past, then started hiking. In the dark. With our flashlights. Single file.

The quiet crunching of hikers ahead and behind created a sense of calm and peace.

Then some noise, heavy panting, loud crunching, "s'cuse me, s'cuse me," as someone flew around us.

We hugged the canyon wall as we heard someone else behind us tripping, sliding, and causing a few rocks to tumble down the canyon. "Hey, watch where you're going!" someone yelled up from further down.

Then we returned to the soft symphony of slow, steady hikers accompanied by the night songs of bugs and brisk breezes brushing through brittle bushes.

We kept a steady but careful pace. Keeping our eyes and flashlights focused on the trail. We glanced up and saw the sky starting to shimmer. Becoming a pale blue as miles and time crept by. We turned one more hairpin switchback and saw two people huddled on the side.

"Are you okay?" I asked.

"Yes," came a woman's raspy voice. "I was going too fast and may have twisted my ankle. My husband is wrapping it. Thanks. We will be fine."

And we were too, until we reached 3 Mile Rest House with a bathroom up the hill and a faucet by the trail. "We still have enough water, so we don't need to fill up until Indian Garden," I said to Rachel. "But this is a good time to eat something. How about a banana? Or part of a PB&J? Or some orange slices?"

Rachel took a small bite of the banana. She chewed, struggled to swallow. "Mom, I just can't eat anything. It feels like my throat is closing up."

What's going on? We had covered our bases, left nothing to chance. Our legs were strong. Our spirits mighty. But Rachel's stomach was weak.

We had not read, heard, or experienced anything like this. I expected lots of lessons on this hike but was stunned we were learning something so soon in the hike. *What have I done? What can I do?* Rachel saw the look in my eyes. Took a few more bites. Gulped hard.

We kept going in the quiet cool and soon entered Indian Garden 4.5 miles from the trailhead. With 50 miles as our goal, I had reviewed the route and listed each milestone and approximate distance. Indian Garden (4.5 miles), Phantom Ranch (13 miles), Cottonwood (19 miles). I calculated the estimated time it would take us on a 3x5 card. So far, we were right on track. We filled our bottles, took a restroom break, glanced up at the towering trees, and passed by the whirring pump station. Eyes glued right.

"There it is, Mom!" Rachel pointed to the tiny Tonto Trailhead sign. We turned right onto the 4+-mile level, meandering interconnecting path. We hit Tip Off in 90 minutes and headed down the steep, stunning South Kaibab Trail.

We traipsed down the trail on our tough, trained legs as cool weather waved goodbye and heat surged up to envelop us. We sipped water and sidelined concerns about Rachel's stomach as she nibbled a few bites and we marveled at the vermillion rocks, verdant bushes, and glittering flecks of golden wildflowers. The trail took us through a dark 20-foot tunnel. When we emerged, the rising sun peaked down over the rim as we stood at the bottom of the Grand Canyon on the bank of the mighty Colorado River.

We tramped across the black suspension bridge, turned left onto a sandy river trail, hung right at the sign, and soon arrived at Phantom Ranch. We were so focused on looking ahead we barely noticed the historic, rustic stone cabins scattered around the little campus. We passed by a large round stone mule train corral and saw the little canteen ahead.

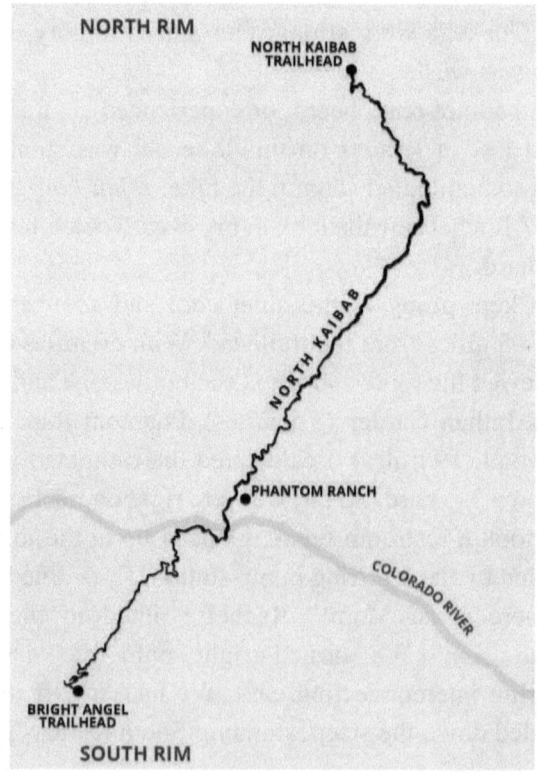

"Rachel, look up! We are surrounded by canyon walls." I chattered more than usual, trying to excite and energize Rachel. Gone were the days when a tiny coin could lift her spirits. There were no shiny dimes on the trail to delight and distract her, but there *were* those brilliant multi-colored layers of rock. Starting with grey at the bottom, the rocks turned a deep plum then a brilliant orange as the towering canyon reached up to greet the sun and touch the bright blue sky.

We sat at a picnic table by the canteen.

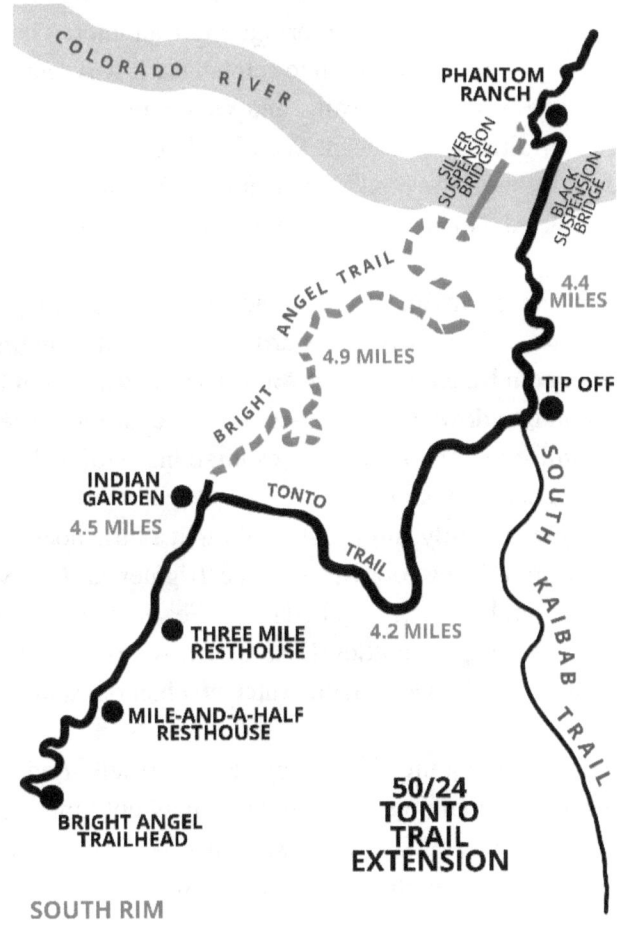

I scrutinized and scratched out numbers on my little card. "We're running about 45 minutes behind my estimated schedule. But I padded in extra time, especially since we don't have to hike those extra miles on the Tonto Trail when we return. I think we're still in good shape to complete in 24 hours. We've already hiked close to 13 miles. We have around 37 miles left. Please try to eat something. Anything, or you'll run out of steam."

"Mom, I feel fine. I'll take a few bites, okay?" She nibbled, gulped, "That's it. Let's go, okay? I'm really scared of the box."

We hiked briskly through the dreaded box canyon, racing the rising sun as we crossed one bridge after another. The spray of Bright Angel Creek floated up to refresh us. It was relatively cool in the shade of the steep walls, and we emerged well before the sun moved directly overhead. We high fived. Rachel exclaimed, "Made it through the box!" It was now 9:00 am, five hours after we had started. Nineteen hours left before our 24-hour completion deadline.

The inner-canyon walls spread out wide, creating an open desert space as we moved forward on the slightly inclining trail from Phantom Ranch to Cottonwood. The sun was out in full force now, pounding down on our hat-covered heads. Our pace slowed. I kept adjusting our milestone estimations, still believing and hoping we could make it.

We met a family, sitting, struggling in a little pocket of shade along the trail. They looked tired and frightened. Overwhelmed with the desert heat. They needed help. We shared our water. Gave them one of our spray bottles. Even better, we gave them the extra bandanas we had soaked with water at Phantom and stuck in a plastic bag.

They were not members of our group. It felt good to be able to offer them something. Wet bandanas may not rank high on the list of awesome gifts, but these folks were delighted. They shouted, "Thank you, thank you!" as we waved and headed down the trail.

We finally saw green up ahead. Our pace had slowed, but we picked it up a bit as we headed into Cottonwood: an oasis with tall trees, a waterspout, picnic tables and restrooms nestled right at the base of the North Rim. Our 24-hour clock was ticking. 11:00 am. Seven hours in. Seventeen hours left.

We sat across from each other on a picnic bench in the shade as we rested and drank. Rachel nibbled a bit more. "Hon, we're an hour and a half behind my schedule and we still have to hike back out. This is our first time and we have already learned some good lessons and know what to expect next time. I don't think we should go any farther."

"Oh Mom, we're so close."

"Not really. We still have more than six miles to the North Rim trailhead."

It hurt to look into Rachel's eyes, still yearning and determined to do the whole thing.

"Can we go just a little farther? You said you were conservative with your milestone times. And once we get to the North Rim, going back downhill will be faster. Please?"

I acknowledged Rachel's compelling rationale and reluctantly agreed.

"Okay," I said. "Let's head up and see how we feel when we get to the bridge."

The hike from Cottonwood to Redwall Bridge was steep. We slowed down. We knew from reading the guidebooks that the trail would become much steeper after the bridge. We crossed at 2:00 p.m. Ten hours from our start. Fourteen hours left. We were running out of time, but just weren't ready to admit it.

We stepped onto the first switchback, sat down on a flat rock, and looked up the daunting trail ahead. Just then, Sid came trotting down the trail and skidded to a stop. "Hi guys!" He paused, cocked his head, "Are you just heading up?"

I slowly nodded yes.

Sid shook his head no.

"It's more than just making it to the top. At your pace it will take you *at least* five hours to get up to the rim and back down to where you are right now. You won't make the 24-hour deadline. And you won't be safe. You decide, but if it were me, I'd turn around now."

Sid adjusted his small pack, started down the trail, then turned.

"Remember, you always have next year."

"He's right, hon," I said.

"I know."

We sat for a while. Rachel took deep breaths, trying not to cry. She wanted this so bad. We gazed at the craggy chasm below Redwall Bridge. Glanced up at the rainbow-colored rocks on the North Rim—and the steep trail that loomed ahead. Then slowly, sadly, packed up our things and headed back down the trail.

Rachel was right. It was much easier descending. By the time we hiked into Cottonwood it was 4:00 p.m. We had been hiking for 12 hours.

Rachel continued to lead. I stopped worrying. Until she started seeing visions in the canyon walls.

"Hey Mom, I see Bert and Ernie in a bathtub. And there's Jean Valjean from *Les Miz*!"

It was nice she remembered seeing *Les Miz*, but she was hallucinating. I got scared.

I walked close behind and kept my eyes glued on her back. Then she stopped and looked down. "Mom, it looks like there are little birds flying in a circle on the path."

I looked down and saw small animal droppings with those nasty big black flies buzzing around.

I prayed. *Please just let us get to Phantom Ranch. Please let Rachel be okay. Please let us find help.*

We hiked into Phantom Ranch at 7:00 p.m. and sat down at the same picnic table where we had stopped that morning. Rachel burst into tears, exhausted, and totally depleted. A hiker filling her bottles at the faucet rushed over when she heard Rachel's sobs. "I remember seeing the two of you at Sid's meeting this morning. What's wrong? Can I help you?"

"My daughter hasn't been able to eat much at all since we started. We had to turn around before getting all the way to the top of North Rim. Now we just need to get out." Then I added so she wouldn't think I was a bad mom, "This never happened before on any of our training hikes. And we did lots of them."

She held up her hand. Took charge.

"Say no more. I have just what she needs. Don't worry, Mom, this happens a lot. For some reason on big hikes like this sometimes your stomach shuts down and it's impossible to eat. I have some protein powder. Give me two of her bottles."

She took a packet of white powder out of her bag and poured some into Rachel's bottles. "Go ahead. Drink this," she commanded as she shook the mixture in one bottle and handed it to Rachel. "It doesn't have any flavor so it will go down easily. Drink it all. Now drink this one too."

I could tell this kind stranger wanted to get going to complete the hike in her best time, but she waited until Rachel had finished both bottles. Then she poured more powder into both. "Wait here for a few more minutes. This should provide enough nutrition for you to get up Bright Angel. You will be fine. Good luck." And she was off.

"Thank you," I called. But she was already way down the trail. I didn't even get her name, but I said a small prayer of thanks in honor of this beautiful bossy stranger.

I didn't know at the time that she would be the first of many *angels* I would meet when I needed them the most, usually on a path.

We sat for a while. Rachel began to perk up. We had to turn around before reaching the North Rim. But now Rachel was stronger. We still had options. "Hon, we can find some place here to sleep on the ground and then hike out whenever we feel strong enough. Or we can go the rest of the way tonight. We even have a little daylight left before turning on our flashlights."

Rachel sat for another minute, considering her choice, growing more resolute. "I want to finish tonight. Let's go."

I heard a trumpet in the recesses of my brain. Then more instruments. The softly stirring theme of *Rocky* started playing in my head.

"Do you still want to lead?"

"Absolutely," she said as she pulled herself together. And off we went.

Out of Phantom Ranch. Across the silver suspension bridge. Along the sandy river trail. My *Rocky*-head-theme was soon accompanied by the rushing roar of the Colorado River. We were marching, climbing, higher and higher.

Rachel set a steady pace. I still hiked closely behind her, watching every step. We reached Devil's Corkscrew. Turned on our flashlights. Slowed a bit. Kept moving forward and upward. The stars twinkled and danced with our flashlight beams as we hiked, finally reaching the plateau. We saw lights up ahead. Lights. Not stars.

And then there were bats.

Some even hit Rachel on the top of her head. This was for real. She was not hallucinating, but I thought I might be. Bats were hitting my daughter's head! And yet she persisted. With tenacity and courage. Brushing them off. Storming forward.

We heard a motor. The Indian Garden pump station! We had made it from Phantom Ranch to Indian Garden in just over two and a half hours. It was 11:00 p.m.

"Rachel, you just led us up from Phantom Ranch at a fast pace, mostly in the dark and even with bats hitting your head. Please always remember how strong you feel right now. You are amazing!" I said as we sat on the wooden bench by the waterspout and a big, beautiful tree. Rachel smiled. She knew. She was clearly proud of herself. Her stomach had relaxed. She could finally eat an entire PB&J. We watched other hikers coming up the trail, murmuring quietly as they filled their bottles, grabbed a quick snack, and headed out.

We were not alone hiking up in the dark, but most of these folks had made it up to the North Rim. And they would complete the full hike in time to earn the right to buy their official R2R2R-50/24 T-shirt. No T-shirts for us this year. No time for regrets. We were safe. Just a bit sad. But also proud.

We headed out on the last portion of the Bright Angel Trail. It was getting cooler. Our bodies were pumping so much heat we did not need our jackets. We headed onward, our flashlights picking up the tiny tunnel about a mile from the top. We seemed to float up that last miracle mile cheered by chirping crickets, embraced by crispy cool air, and greeted by welcoming lights scattered along the South Rim, celebrating our return. It was 2:30 am. Twenty-two and a half hours after we had started.

Now we were cold and sore. We hobbled on our chilled, stiffening legs and plopped into the car. It was hard to drive with the fog outside on the road and inside my head, but we finally made it to Kaibab Lodge. We looked around for the deer we had seen yesterday morning. Sad not to see him. Not sure why. After spending another minute searching, we slowly, painfully dragged ourselves up the steps to our room.

After a few hours of restless sleep, we hauled ourselves out of bed, exhausted but determined not to miss the festive finish breakfast at El Tovar. Even if we didn't make it all the way we deserved to celebrate. We had some blisters, a few wobbly toenails, and spectacularly sore muscles. Our pride was injured, but not our resolve. We gingerly hobbled down the stairs, muscles throbbing and screaming with every step.

Sid's face lit up when we walked into the crowded dining room. "You made it! So glad you could join us!" he said with a big smile and a hint of relief.

We found a table and ordered our breakfast, a big one, consisting of softly scrambled eggs (yellow, not brown), golden, crispy hash browns, short stacks drenched in syrup, and toast smothered with strawberry jam. We earned it. Every bite.

The *Arizona Highways* journalist, William Hafford, walked up to our table.

"Hi there, may I sit with you for a few minutes? I've been interviewing folks who completed the hike. Sid told me the two of you didn't make it the whole way, but he was sure you had a great story to tell. You're the only mother-daughter team and you both look great this morning. It looks like you worked up quite an appetite," he grinned. "So can you tell me about your experience?" We gave him the highlights, especially about the anonymous hiker angel who gave Rachel the protein powder.

He kept shaking his head.

"And so here you are," he said. "You hiked at least 45 miles, did not complete the full event, and yet you're still smiling. I sprained my ankle and didn't even make it to Phantom Ranch, so I get it. We hiked the Grand Canyon and there's always next year. Right?" He started to move on, then turned around. "You must be very proud of your daughter, and yourself. Good job." He smiled and headed over to another table.

When the *Arizona Highways* article came out the following February, he included portions of his interview with us, concluding with, "Although they didn't finish their rim crossing, Rachel and her mother had spent more than 22 hours hiking on the trail, nearly 10 of them in darkness."

On our way back to the car, we stopped at the patio behind Bright Angel Lodge and gazed at the canyon. We could trace the slice across the bottom where we had hiked.

We asked someone to take our picture. It would be the first of many pictures of us through the years standing in that same place, always smiling, always safe. Not always successful, but still able to savor sweet stories of hiking the Grand Canyon.

I had read about archivists restoring a piece of art, then noticing a chip in the top layer and discovering a spectacular painting in the layer below. That's kind of what happened to us. At first, our adventure was hidden under a lackluster gray saga of *did not complete*.

But, every time we shared our story, we chipped off another piece of that gray to see something new and beautiful about our experience. We began to recognize how much we had accomplished and how we had been transformed by all that happened and all we learned.

Rachel and I had hiked almost 45 miles down, across and up the Grand Canyon, in daylight and dark, with joy and sadness, strong legs, mighty spirits, and weak stomachs. We turned around to be safe. We helped a family be safe with water and wet bandanas. We received support from a stranger. We weren't injured. We were inspired. Something new and exciting had become embedded in our souls.

Our fear of failure did not disappear but was certainly diminished. Our courage and curiosity increased. We continued to train hard and push ourselves. We also became more willing to participate in challenging events, even those with an element of risk and no guarantee of success.

We didn't fully understand the impact on our lives at the time, but we did recognize that taking risks and stepping into the unknown was the right choice for us.

Many years later when I looked back on my life map pondering all the new trails I had taken, new places I had explored, new challenges I had embraced since walking into that writing class when I was 45, I saw how this first adventure was a big deal. I had left a secure job. Studied for a new academic challenge. And started on a quest to hike 50 miles in the Grand Canyon by the time I turned 50.

I was moving forward with no clear picture of where this new path would take me, but I was no longer bored or stuck. I wondered if I ever would be again. I *was* curious, scared, and excited to see what was waiting round the bend. I was also sure that, no matter what, I would always remember this was the point when my life had been changed for good. And maybe Rachel's too.

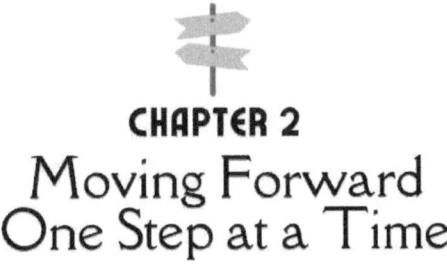

CHAPTER 2
Moving Forward
One Step at a Time

Rachel and I failed to complete the Grand Canyon hike. I had not scored high enough on the GMAT. I was almost 50 years old.

Was this all that was waiting round the bend for me?

No.

Quitting was not an option. Working harder was. Learning more too. So that's what I did.

I took Algebra 1 since I had forgotten most of what I had learned a million years ago in my high school freshman class. Then Algebra 2. Then Advanced Algebra/trig.

And finally, after a year of studying, it was GMAT #2 showtime. I got up early, exercised in our living room to my Jane Fonda video so I could fill my brain with oxygen. (I had read that it helped.) Ate a healthy breakfast. Then sniffed some cinnamon to calm me down. (Read that too.) I drove to the U of A campus and walked back into the test center, sharpened pencils clutched in my hand, and armed with a full year of preparation, practice, and study, I knew what I had to do.

And this time I did it! I scored well into the 90th percentile and was accepted into the September 1991 Management and Policy doctoral program at the University of Arizona.

I soon learned that getting in the program was just the first hurdle. My advisor, Dr. Lee Beach, offered a warm welcome along with a candid warning, "Sandi, you are not our typical PhD student. You're older with years of experience and we plan to take full advantage of your business and community leadership skills by fulfilling your TA responsibilities with teaching assignments throughout your entire program. That will be the easy part. The harder part will be your classwork and RA assignments where you stop thinking like a manager and start thinking like a researcher. This will be totally new for you. Later you'll be able to combine all your abilities and knowledge, but your first year will be hard."

It was.

I had to prove myself, especially since I did not earn stellar grades in my classes that first year. So, I volunteered to support additional research projects. Edited a manuscript for one of the professors. Served as student advisor and helped design a management course that I co-taught with a full professor. Kris, a young peer, helped me navigate statistics that first year. Suzanne Cummins, a lawyer and one of the new instructors who knew Arnie from Little League, encouraged and supported me, becoming a lifelong friend.

Gradually other professors recognized I could add value to the program. One told me a few years later, "It took you a bit longer than the younger students to get up to speed, but once we saw you in action, it was hard to ignore or discount your determination and results. Your maturity and leadership brought a great deal to the classes you taught, and your research too. I'm glad you toughed it out." So was I.

And I continued my quest to hike the Grand Canyon R2R2R 50/24 by the time I turned 50.

Rachel and I treated our first 50/24 as a beginning and immediately started training for 1992. We reserved early this year and got a room at Bright Angel Lodge right on the South Rim. We had tested all kinds of nutrition products and eating approaches so we and our stomachs would be ready for our second hike. We learned that eating high-carb meals starting a few days before the hike helped us to digest more carbs the night before. Bagels with cream cheese became our best friend in the morning.

We were ready. But apparently not everyone else was. Sid had sent an email saying the hike had been cancelled. Then

36

another email saying the hike was still on, but it would be informal, not official. Our confusion increased, but our commitment didn't waver. In May 1992, we drove to the Canyon, a bit concerned by the emails, but totally confident this would be our year to complete the 50/24, from rim to rim to rim.

It wasn't. While we were in control of ourselves, we could not control the universe.

Bright Angel Lodge lobby was filled with hikers, just like last year. Sid was already standing in his usual place on the hearth of the giant fireplace. But nothing else was the same. It was quiet, subdued, no cheerful chattering. He called everyone together. A tall man stood close by his side. In a uniform. Scowling.

Sid started talking, his voice uncharacteristically flat. "Welcome everyone. A few things have changed this year, so let me start with the easy part. The trail to the North Rim has been closed for repairs. We will not be able to hike our usual 50/24. We have mapped out a detour hike from Phantom Ranch to Clear Creek. This hike will be shorter, 40 miles, but will be just as challenging, maybe even harder due to the heat on this portion of the canyon. We will hike but it will not be the same."

After the moaning and groaning subsided, Sid continued, "And we have a bigger problem that may affect the future of this hike all together."

The National Park Service representative stepped forward, scrunched his face into an even deeper scowl, and announced, "We no longer support this event. If you persist, we may treat this as a criminal act. If you walk out to the trailhead after this meeting, we will video your face and record your name and address."

This warning and approach seemed so heavy-handed that most of us neglected to even try to understand the rationale for the change. NPS had reluctantly supported this event in the early years, but after the *Arizona Highways* article hit the stands, they feared the worst: that the group would become too big and unmanageable, dangerous to the canyon and to other hikers.

The representative continued, "When people explore the canyon in small groups, they take care of themselves and each other. When there's a crowded competitive event like this, it's every man for himself. Some folks lose their common sense, and we are left to pick up the pieces."

"Consider yourselves warned," he growled as he stepped off the hearth and headed to the Bright Angel trailhead, joining a small group armed with notepads, bright lights, and video equipment.

We were so ready! We had done everything we could to make sure we could complete the entire hike this year. I turned to Rachel. "I'm bummed enough that the North Rim trail is closed, but the worst part is I might turn you into a criminal!"

Rachel wiped her tears. "I know we could do the whole thing this year. I'm more frustrated about the route change than that guy's threats. They're just going to video us right now, not arrest us. We're not convicts. Not yet! Let's do it."

We saw the bright lights and video equipment. Appropriately intimidating. I struggled to ignore that judgy voice accusing me of being a bad mom, leading my daughter onto a path of crime. It was eerily quiet except for the interrogations. Our resolve weakened, but our feet kept moving forward. We faced the camera. Squinted in the blinding lights. Gave our name and address. Then started slowly down the trail.

We watched the flashlights sparkle on the dark trail as we hiked in a subdued procession, more funerary than fun. No stampeding runners passing us this time. That was the one nice change.

Our pace was good. We both felt strong as we opened ourselves up to the majestic canyon. We celebrated milestone memories from last year's hike: first tunnel, second tunnel, 1.5 Mile Resthouse. We stepped off the trail at 3 Mile Resthouse to grab snacks from our packs. Rachel's stomach happily cooperated this year as we munched on bananas and split our first PB&J.

We were heartened, gradually gaining confidence and speed as we nimbly hiked down Jacob's Ladder and onto the rocky path leading into Indian Garden. Rachel walked ahead stalwart and strong.

I marched behind my happy, confident daughter. Light on my feet. I even started to jog. Then suddenly my bubble of joy popped as my left foot jammed into a pothole. "Agh!!"

"Rachel, stop! Something happened to my foot."

She spun around and stared as I tried to keep walking. I took a step downhill. My foot felt squishy, like nothing was holding it together.

Rachel took a deep breath. Tried to put on a brave face, but she was crushed.

"Are you sure, Mom? You can't go any further?"

Took a few more steps. Felt more mush. "I'm sure."

"What do we do now?" Rachel fought back her tears.

"Let me tighten my boot and see if I can hike uphill. I am so sorry."

We reluctantly turned around on another Grand Canyon hike and started the slow climb back up the 4.3 miles to the rim. My foot hurt, but since we were hiking uphill, I could keep the pressure on my heels and off my toes.

"I'm old enough to know better," I muttered. "What in this whole wide world made me think I could run in the Grand Canyon? I can't even run on level ground!"

We reached the beautiful boulder shelter at 3 Mile Resthouse and sat on one of the wooden benches surrounding the shaded perimeter. No need to hurry. No big hike to complete. We filled our water bottles and chatted with other hikers who were on their way down. Most were new to the canyon, filled with questions, somewhat unprepared. It felt good to provide updates, encouragement, and answers. Rachel looked a little less sad as we helped these other hikers, even giving them most of our trail snacks since we no longer needed them.

We headed out from the resthouse. I couldn't delight Rachel with dimes on the trail, but I kept searching for a silver lining.

"You know what, Rachel? My foot is so swollen that my boot is doing double duty as a cast holding all that spongy tissue together."

She stopped, turned, and gave me a look, knowing full well what I was doing and what I was about to say. "Go ahead, Mom. Say it."

"How fortuitous!"

She shook her head, smiled, started hiking again with a tiny bounce to her step as we gradually moved up the trail, now bathed in sunlight. Then Rachel discovered her own shiny perspective. "Mom, this is our first time hiking this trail in daylight."

"You're right! What a beautiful sight," I agreed. The canyon echoed our dawning joy, calling out, "Look at me!" as we hiked around another switchback. We stopped and looked down, able to see all the way to the snaking trail surrounded by yellow brush and grey rocks, slithering into the green oasis of Indian Garden. We arrived at the South Rim, not gleeful by any means, but with our spirits a bit brighter. The sun was more friendly on the rim than it would be along the bottom.

When we finally made it back to the cabin, I took off my boot and sock. Gasped as this foreign multi-colored gelatinous mass oozed out. I called Arnie sobbing. "Hon. You're going to be okay. There's a hospital on the South Rim. Go there. Get some help. I love you."

We drove to the tiny Grand Canyon Hospital just a few miles away. The doctor gazed at my misshaped appendage in wonder. "You were able to hike all the way back from Indian Garden on this? It's a mess. But the X-ray doesn't show anything is broken, so it must just be a nasty sprain. The only thing I can do is wrap it with an Ace bandage and give you some crutches. Try to stay off your foot as much as possible."

Later that night, we posed for our second-year picture with

the unconquered canyon behind us, still beaconing, urging us to try again next year.

We joined some hikers for breakfast at El Tovar, shared our saga, and heard stories from many others who had not completed the adjusted hike. Some turned back due to the extreme heat. Some hiked the wrong way and had to backtrack. A few who had hiked the entire way to Clear Creek in the blazing sun barely made it back. One hiker slept along the Bright Angel Trail most of the night suffering from heat exhaustion. He had just hiked out with the help of his friend a few hours earlier.

Sid and the rest of the organizers were determined to make the best of it. "If you showed up this year, you have earned the right to buy this year's specially designed T-shirt," (which I still have) Sid said. "I'm not sure what the future of this hike will be now that the Park Service is treating us like outlaws. But at this point, we plan to continue to train and hike around the same time next year. We will just stay under the radar, hike in smaller groups of 2 or 3, and start out between 3:00 and 4:00 am, not all at the same time."

First R2R2R 50/24 attempt: May 1991. Did not finish.

Second R2R2R 50/24 alternative attempt: May 1992. Broke the law. Broke my foot. Spirit still intact.

My passion for the R2R2R 50/24 had not abated. I was 48. Two more years until 1994, the year I would turn 50. I had to achieve this feat by then or give it up.

But at this point, Rachel had better things to do.

On one of our evening walks, Rachel said, "Mom, I'm not giving up on the 50/24. I still want to go on some walks and hikes with you, just don't want to go through all the training. Maybe put it on hold until I finish high school."

"I completely understand, hon. I'll keep training and hiking to meet my goal, but we have the rest of our lives to complete our hike together." (At this point I didn't realize how many years, even decades that would take.)

My frustration healed quickly. My foot not so much. After six months of pain, I finally went to a podiatrist. "I sprained my foot last May when I hiked the Grand Canyon. It just doesn't seem like it's getting much better. It still hurts a lot."

She nodded while she looked at the X-ray of my foot. "When did you get that stress fracture across the base of your toes? All I see is a bunch of scar tissue, so there's nothing I can do about the break. But that's probably what's been causing you all this pain."

I was stunned. "They X-rayed my foot at the Grand Canyon and said nothing was broken."

"Your foot was probably so swollen the stress fracture didn't show up. It happens in cases like this. I can make some orthotics for you. Maybe a firmer shoe might help alleviate some of the pain. I'm guessing you're not going to give up on this quest, right?"

"Right."

I continued to train, doing more walking and hiking with my dear friends Ann Galloway and Carole Sheehan. Ann and I had been friends since second grade. In many ways she was the only person outside my family who shared my childhood memories. We shared a history. We sorted things out from our past, encouraged each other, and helped each other as we walked up and down the 7.4-mile tram route at Sabino Canyon.

Later she told me, "If it hadn't been for you and your crazy R2R2R 50/24 determination, I would never have even attempted that 100-mile biking event. You are a great influence on me!"

Carole and I had known each other for about ten years. I had introduced her to the joy of long walking. Later, she was delighted to do many of the even longer, steeper training hikes with me.

Of course, every walk and hike became much more than just training for a big event. My friendship with both women grew much deeper as we shared those many miles together. Walking friendships were becoming part of my newly transformed life.

One year later, even though Rachel had decided to skip the

hike, she still wanted to drive up to the canyon with me and hang out on the South Rim while I hiked. She could relax and explore some of the rim trails.

Since this was no longer a formal event, I started alone at 3:00 a.m. for my third R2R2R 50/24 attempt. We had turned around just before Indian Garden when I broke my foot last year, so this would be my second hike across Tonto Trail, down South Kaibab to Phantom Ranch, pick up North Kaibab, hike through the box, across the bottom, into Cottonwood, and up the North Rim. It was fun getting reacquainted with the trail, noticing little things I had missed during our first crossing. I also reminded myself of my new lesson regarding jogging. Never again. Not for me. Ever.

My head was clear, pace good, legs strong, but both feet were busy building blisters—probably due to the inflexible orthotics and different shoes I was wearing. By the time I reached the little 3-mile sign on the North Rim trail after hiking almost 23 miles, I knew it was time to stop, turn around and hike back out. I would not finish. Again.

This should have been totally devastating, but it wasn't. How could that be?

Because.

In that moment, I *knew* I had to turn around. My body told me so. In a quiet voice that softly announced, "It's time."

You have about 20 miles left in you. Turn back now.

I listened. I turned around.

The beauty of this moment was that through my failures to complete I had internalized a wealth of information about me: my stamina, my being. I had become smarter, better, stronger.

And I still had one more year to complete the entire hike by the time I turned 50!

I felt confident, ready to hike back out. There were blisters on my blisters, but my feet were the *only* problem this time. I liked the way I felt, mentally and physically, as I retraced my steps back down to Cottonwood, across the canyon bottom, to Phantom Ranch, over the silver bridge, and up Devil's Corkscrew.

I approached two women who had hiked down to Phantom that morning and were struggling as they slowly slogged their way back up. They were surprised at how much harder it was to hike *up* Bright Angel. It happens.

I stayed with them for a short while to reassure them and make sure they were okay. They had flashlights and enough water. I gave them more snacks. Then headed on up, knowing my body would soon start to flag.

It was dark by the time I heard the welcoming sound of the Indian Garden pump station. I arrived at about the same time Rachel and I did two years ago. Memories surrounded me. Thankfully, no bats.

Almost home! Just 4.5 miles left. Up, up, up I went, feeling the slow steady drain of my remaining energy, happy I had turned around when I did. I trudged up Bright Angel delighted at the burst of energy as I hiked up the final switchback.

"Did you make it?" Rachel sleepily asked when I opened our cabin door.

"No, my blisters got the best of me, but I'm fine. I finished strong and there's always next year. Go back to sleep. I'll tell you all about it tomorrow morning. There's no breakfast at El Tovar this year so we can sleep as late as we want."

We enjoyed a post-hike breakfast of eggs, hashbrowns, pancakes, and toast at Bright Angel Lodge, then walked out to the patio for picture number three with the Grand Canyon and North Rim looming in the distance.

Third R2R2R 50/24 attempt, May 1993. Blisters—yes. Body smart—yes. Body strong—oh yes!

Some folks just could not understand. "Why don't you just take a shorter hike and enjoy the scenery? How can hiking more than 50 miles in 24 hours be fun or even reasonable? Perhaps even responsible? Is the T-shirt that important? This is crazy! You are crazy!"

But I loved the entire process, training, pushing myself, hiking with friends and family, hiking alone. Basking in beautiful nature. Shooting for an audacious goal. A motivating goal. It pushed me and pulled me. Kept me fit. Made me happy.

Hiking across the Grand Canyon was embedded in my soul. I refused to shake my dream.

Although, occasionally I wavered. Just a bit.

I headed out alone one morning to hike a small section of one of my favorite Sabino trails along Esperero Canyon. It was one of the few times I had hiked a side trail alone and was delighted to meet another woman headed the same direction. We clicked and hiked together. She told me about her life as a snowbird, her love of hiking, spending nine months in Tucson and the rest of the year back in Michigan.

I told her my R2R2R 50/24 story. "Many of us slow hikers don't have much time to sit and enjoy the scenery, but it's still a beautiful experience. Crossing the Grand Canyon from one rim to the other and back again is simply a dream I can't shake. It's firmly lodged in my head and heart."

I continued, "During my last attempt, I had hiked almost 23 miles before turning around. And in that final stretch up the South Rim after being on the trail for more than 40 miles, something magical happened. The stars, night sounds, and elevation change. My exhaustion turned to exhilaration. When I reached trail's end, my sense of euphoria was overwhelming. I can't describe the depth of feeling of those final hours, leaving almost every ounce of energy on the trail. Totally depleted. I just *loved* it.

"Next year I will go the whole way. I need to. Is this crazy? Does this even make sense?"

We hiked together. Same pace. In synch. She listened, nodded, and seemed to understand my turmoil even though we had just met. "Well, it's not crazy to you," she said. "And it makes sense to you. And you want to do this. So, I think you already have your answer."

She continued, "But maybe you can give your quandary the rocking chair test. When you are too old to do much of anything except rock in your chair and review your past, will it make you happy to think about this time in your life? Will you be glad you persevered and continued chasing this dream? Will you celebrate your accomplishment when you finally complete the entire hike? Or will it make you happy to think that you quit chasing this dream and did something less crazy and more reasonable?"

Clearly this woman was profoundly credible. She was a hiker. She hadn't burst out laughing when I asked her advice. And she told me exactly what I needed to hear.

She heard my question and understood my quest. We both knew my need to do the R2R2R 50/24 passed the rocking chair test.

I didn't know this woman, don't even remember her name. Yet I was willing to take the chance, ask her advice, and listen to her answer. I learned that the wisdom of strangers can make a big difference. I didn't realize it then, but chance encounters with strangers would continue to enhance my life in all the years to come. Later, I included them in my growing list of angels.

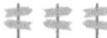

1994 came around. This was it. I had turned 50 in February. Learned my lessons. Worked harder. Bought better shoes and socks. Ditched the orthotics. Did not quit. This was my year. Rachel rode up to the canyon with me again, both of us confident I would make it. We bought our traditional *50 Beautiful Most People In The World* issue of People Magazine, this time with Meg Ryan on the cover.

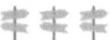

There was no morning meeting and just a few others on the

trail when I headed out at 4:00 a.m. Rachel walked me to the trail, gave me a big hug, and headed back to the cabin to sleep. And I was off, secure, strong, and profoundly happy to renew acquaintance with my grand friend.

Each milestone brought memories and confidence. 3 Mile Resthouse, Indian Garden, pump station, and the little Tonto Trail sign on the right. Familiar and comfortable. I sailed (but did not jog) across Tonto. I hiked fast, safe, secure. Turned left and headed down South Kaibab across the black suspension bridge, happily stopping at Phantom Ranch to eat a PB&J. I gazed up at the blue ribbon of sky shimmering above the inner canyon walls.

It was another 100+ degree day across the bottom. I was prepared. My pace was steady. Through Cottonwood, up North Rim trail, past Roaring Springs, over Redwall Bridge, and up the switchbacks—all 27 of them. No turning back this time. Legs strong. Lungs fighting for air. Climbing steep and strong. North Rim trailhead. Made it!

Chilly. Snowy patches on the ground. Had to move fast. I quickly found someone to take my picture as I draped myself over the trailhead sign, lifting my right thumb up. (A funny picture. I looked a little loopy. Probably was.) I gobbled a snack, fighting the chill, then headed right back down the trail, ending up leapfrogging and then chatting with the same hiker who had taken my picture on the rim. We kept each other company until Cottonwood where he reconnected with the rest of his party who were also quietly doing the *unofficial* 50/24.

There were few others on the trail, but I never felt alone. I heard someone hiking behind me most of the way. When I turned into Phantom, he called out, "Good job! You were a great pacer for me." (I was a pacer for someone else?! Astonishing.)

I ate another BP&J at Phantom Ranch, filled my water bottles, and headed out, over the silver bridge and up, making great time. Heard that familiar friendly welcoming whirring sound of the Indian Garden pump station.

It started to get chilly shortly after leaving Indian Garden, so I stopped to put on my lightweight jacket and sit on an inviting flat rock. I could finally allow myself to acknowledge that after three attempts, I was just about to capture my goal of hiking the entire R2R2R 50/24 at 50. I was strong and invincible. Helen Reddy's song, "I Am Woman," echoed in my head. I hugged myself. Hard.

Then I saw a flashlight beam as another hiker came clomping up the trail. "Hi, are you okay? I'm guessing you are part of the 50/24 group. Did you make it the whole way?" he asked.

"I'm fine and yes, after years of training and learning, and three attempts, I finally made it."

"Congratulations! I completely missed the Tonto Trail turnoff. By the time I realized it, I had gone too far to turn back so I hiked to the bottom and took the side trip to Ribbon Falls. There's always next year to complete the whole thing. My name is Mike. Do you want to hike up this last part together? I like to keep a slow, steady pace so I don't have to stop and catch my breath."

"I'm Sandi. Hiking together sounds great. Thank you. Please take the lead."

We hiked slowly and steadily up Jacob's Ladder. Just before 3 Mile Resthouse, we saw someone hunched over by the side of the trail. "Would you like to join us?" Mike asked.

He sounded young, tired, and scared. "I'd love to." The three of us trudged single file up Bright Angel. Mike offered observations, told stories, shared historical tidbits. His deep voice droned, accompanied by the soft night chorus of crickets and scurrying critters.

As we neared the trailhead, the sound of Mike's voice receded. I heard the soft strains of "Hallelujah," faintly familiar, profoundly touching. My chest tightened. My eyes burned. I struggled to breathe as we reached the end. Not fatigued. My heart and lungs were filled with joy.

We emerged into the soft quiet of the South Rim at 1:10 am, 21 hours and 50 minutes after I had started the morning before. Mike turned to me in the dark and said, "Congratulations, Sandi. You did it!"

"Thank you! And it only took five years of dreaming, training, and learning, plus three attempts," I laughed. We parted ways, never seeing each other's faces, but grateful for the sweet connection. (Later I would meet him in daylight at a 50/24 "reunion." And even later we would meet again when I became his matchmaker.)

I approached our cabin, opened the door. "I knew you'd do it!" Rachel jumped up out of bed and hugged me, not even asking if I had. She could see it all in my smile. She had stayed up and left the lights on for me. Of course.

I finally met my Grand Canyon goal.

At the end of 1995, five years after I left the telephone company, I took a moment to ponder my/our decision to take that 5+5 buy-out. I remembered the facilitator of the transition workshop asking us to describe what the next five years would bring. Most of what I wrote back then came true. We all grew older. Our lives were enhanced, reinvented.

However, I did not know my mom would die suddenly of a heart attack shortly before she turned 80. I had not been able to say goodbye to her, which was devastating. I was delighted with how we had spent those final precious years of her life, but I struggled to fill the void. The hole in my heart. The profound loss. I felt broken. *When will it stop hurting so much? How can I cope?*

I couldn't even say goodbye!

Gradually, hiking helped me heal. One day at Sabino Canyon, I stopped at Bridge 5 on the tram route to toss a stone into the bubbling stream. I remembered how Mom brought me and my brother Chuck here to dig for sand rubies in the beach by the water. Later, she brought Rachel and Jonathan to the same place. It was here she introduced us to the delight of discovering shiny treasures in nature. I realized she would always be with me, especially outside, on a trail, in my heart.

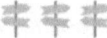

One evening Rachel sat down with us after dinner. "I know I should go to college. I also know I'm not ready and would just waste your money and my time. I've decided to join the military," she said with that same look of determination she had when we sat at the picnic table at Phantom Ranch. She knew what she needed to do, understood it would be hard, was willing to embrace the scary unknown.

Jonathan started high school and joined the wrestling team. During the summers, Arnie chauffeured him to roller hockey, ice hockey, even karate. And he joined me on my visits to the Tucson *eegee's* restaurants where I administered questionnaires to the hourly workers and interviewed managers for my dissertation research.

Arnie went back to college, explored a whole new world of learning, and earned a BS in Business Administration. He started working full time. We took conference trips and discovered the delight of exploring fascinating cities right here in the U.S.

Our years were filled with sunny days and calm breezes most of the time. We also had our share of marital maelstroms and teenager turbulence as we explored our new path. There were high peaks, deep valleys, and even a few instances of feeling like we were falling into an abyss. When we were totally lost, we relied on counselors to help us get back on track. We made it though, older, wiser, always together, stronger, more resilient, more committed to build on lessons learned and to adjust missteps.

I completed my course work and wrote a thesis in my minor,

earning a MS in Higher Ed Administration. Then passed my doctoral written exam, orals, and defended my dissertation on the work demands and controls of a young, diverse population of fast-food workers. I presented my findings to the members of my committee, then stepped out of the room to sit in the hall while they deliberated. After about fifteen minutes, my dissertation chair opened the door, walked out, smiled, reached out her hand and said, "Congratulations, Dr. Richmond."

Dr. Beach came out last and walked me down the hall. "For the next few weeks every time any of us sees you, we will make it a point to greet you as *Dr. Richmond*. It's what we do to get you used to your new title, so you don't start giggling every time you hear it," he laughed.

And that's exactly what happened. "Good morning, Dr. Richmond. Good afternoon, Dr. Richmond. Nice to see you Dr. Richmond."

I continued to hike at least a portion of the cross-canyon trail once a year until it was time to leave Tucson, yet I never completed it in the *exact* way to qualify for another official R2R2R-50/24 T-shirt. Mostly I hiked with Carole, sometimes other friends. We tried different starting times, different months of the year, and finally cut out the extra Tonto Trail miles, heading straight down the Bright Angel Trail to hike a *regular* R2R2R.

One time we hiked across the bottom during a full moon, so brilliant we could turn off our flashlights. The moon's luminescent glow transformed the inner canyon walls, rocks, even the desert grasses into glass-like formations. It felt like we were walking through a sparkling crystal palace.

And then it came time to move on—out of Tucson, away from the Grand Canyon, and into a new job on the opposite side of the country.

Kris, the young PhD student who had helped me at the beginning of my program, had started working in Orlando at Walt Disney World a few years earlier. He described me to his director who then recruited me. My former boss and mentor at US West, Ruel Cooper, wrote one of my reference letters. So did Dr. Beach and Suzanne Cummins, who I now count as dear friends.

On a Saturday morning in June 1998, I sat on a rock chatting with Carole at Cardiac Gap on the ridge of Esperero Trail. (That same trail where I met the *rocking chair* hiker.) "It's hard to believe we won't be spending any more Saturday mornings hiking up here now that you're moving to Florida," said Carole as we munched on chunks of her homemade banana bread.

"I agree," I said. "This is a great career opportunity. It's just tough to leave Tucson."

Carole reminisced, "Way back when you first left the phone company you were terrified. But you made the right decision and it all worked out. And you changed my life too! It's obvious that taking big risks and jumping into the unknown is a good lifestyle for you and those around you."

I laughed, remembering how I had changed her life. "We were shooting for your first official R2R2R 50/24 back in 1996 but we ended up taking more than 30 hours. We had climbed up to the North Rim trailhead and were almost back to Phantom Ranch when we had to stop and rest by the trail because your ankle was so sore from rubbing on your boot. You slept. I sat and listened to the nighttime cricket sounds in the dark. There was a brief silence. Then bird songs heralded a new day at first light. It was another magical Grand Canyon moment I'll never forget."

I stayed with that memory for a moment as Carole continued by sharing her magical moment when she first met Mike, "And I'll never forget meeting Mike. We were sitting on the rocks by the final bridge in the box when he came around the corner, looking frustrated. He told us he got sick and had to turn around again. You introduced us and told him about my injured foot."

"There were certainly some sparks between the two of you that day," I smiled. "He helped you climb up and out, and the rest is history." (She and Mike eventually got married. At the Grand

Canyon. Of course).

The bags and boxes were packed. We were ready to go. We said farewell to the people and places that had been part of our lives. I hiked the R2R2R one more time, saying goodbye and savoring all the sweetness of those many years on these canyon trails and how my life had changed.

I learned it doesn't matter how hard it is at the beginning; it can get easier, with diligence, determination, luck, and the goodness of others. Working hard and moving fast is good as long as I don't overdo it and hit a pothole. And when I do hit a pothole, I learn and do better the next time.

Through all these years, there were many reasons to quit. Too hard. Too much. Unsafe. Unknown. Unrealistic. Crazy. But there were no *valid* reasons. For me. That is what I will remember. I spent these years, trusting myself, trusting Arnie—leaning on him, embracing family, friends, even strangers, gathering information, getting stronger, and learning more about my body, my mind, my dreams, my priorities.

I now knew how I wanted to live my life and who I wanted to be going forward.

CHAPTER 3
Milepost 55:
Discovering New Paths

I can see my breath, but not my feet. I'm shivering in a corral heaving with humanity. It's 5:30 am, January 8, 2000. The start of a new decade and a brand-new experience. I'm getting ready to walk my first marathon, the Walt Disney World Marathon. Off in the distance Mickey Mouse is waving his white-gloved hand standing on top of a lighted arch.

How did I end up here? Why aren't I terrified?

Last July, I received an email announcing that Walt Disney World (WDW) Cast Members could participate in the WDW Marathon for free. And it was walker friendly! What a wonderful opportunity to try something new, especially since Arizona and the Grand Canyon were so far away. All I had to do was learn what was involved in walking a marathon, start training, and find a partner.

I wanted to share this amazing experience, so I spent weeks asking friends and colleagues to join me in this event. Most people were not nearly as enthusiastic as I was about this opportunity as I was. (Interesting.) Finally, one of my peers, Kathy, said yes.

So here we are. My heart is pounding, and we haven't even started walking. There are dozens of other women in their 50s and 60s participating in this event. Most of them are *real* athletes—runners, standing in corrals far ahead of ours.

For some reason I'm not frightened even though I've never done anything like this before. I'm a tad worried we won't walk fast enough to avoid getting swept. Like she's reading my mind, Kathy asks, "Do you think we'll be fast enough to stay ahead of the sweeper?"

I need to reassure her (and myself). "Trust me, I've done all the calculations. We're good."

Kathy is 13 years younger than I, but I'm the recruiter, leader, time tracker, and motivator of our little team of two.

Earlier in the month, I did my homework, learned the route, and figured at our average 15-minute-per-mile pace, we could walk the 26.2 miles in a little more than six and a half hours. Tight but doable.

We have 10 minutes until the official start of the race. It will take around another 5-10 minutes for our corral to inch up to the start line, so I just chill, literally and figuratively. Epcot Tapestry of Nations music provides background to the chatter around me.

"Kathy," I say. "I just overheard that most participants are planning to toss their warm-up sweats and jackets to the side of the corral when we start. Then volunteers pick them up and donate them to homeless shelters. How cool! Next year, we can be comfy warm in our extra layers, then help someone else be warm long after the marathon is over."

I know there are water stops, but I still wear a little fanny pack with staples from my Grand Canyon hikes—a PB&J and supersized package of peanut M&M's. I also carry a small bottle of water to get me to the first water station.

The minutes tick by. Then silence. The loudspeaker stops blaring. Mickey Mouse stands still. We hear the national anthem. Then, a gunshot. Racers in wheelchairs in the corral to our left head out. Now that is courageous!

Our corral compresses. Distance between participants evaporates. A bit claustrophobic. Thank goodness Kathy and I are both tall. Another gunshot and we can see runners ahead of us begin. Five minutes later we start moving. It's slow going until we get close to the START arch. We finally cross the timing pad.

Our group remains congested. Then runners forge ahead. Walkers spread out. We pick up our pace, passing others, many of whom are dressed in costumes. What a surprise. I expected to see fancy running clothes but never dreamed we would see a dinosaur costume or Micky and Minnie outfits. We come up behind a bride in white and a groom in black with the guts to tackle 26.2 miles wearing a short bridal veil and tall top hat.

There goes Ariel with her mermaid tail flopping behind! Here comes Snow White in a short skirt running with a dwarf—"Happy," of course. Ballerinas in pink tutus. Supermen in blue tights. Outfits in all styles and colors of the rainbow represented. Oh wait, there's someone dressed in rainbow colors with a huge arc over their head!

We weave in and out among slower walkers and pass by the first mile marker in 13 minutes. Our weekly training hikes are paying off. Only 25.2 miles to go!

We wind through Epcot, walk by Spaceship Earth, then head out and around the back of the park passing Mile Markers 2, 3, and 4. Our pace is brisk as we walk in the quiet cool morning. We leave Epcot and its big wide world behind, turn right onto World Drive, and head toward Magic Kingdom with its Small, Small World. A soft breeze refreshes us. The rising sun brightens the sky.

We pass a few more mile markers fast, strong, and steady. I relax.

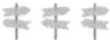

My mind wanders back to 1998 when I was recruited by the WDW Organization Development director, Chris King, to join his young internal consulting team.

He appreciated my experience, my age, even my graying hair. Figured older leaders might feel comfortable with me even though I would be an outsider. The job sounded intriguing. The timing was good.

Working at Walt Disney World could be a wonderful new experience, but the location would be awful. "Florida is humid. Florida is flat. There are *no* mountains," I told Arnie.

"That's true, hon," Arnie said as he sat down and opened an atlas, "but we'd be near the ocean and the East Coast. It would be an adventure. Worth a try. Especially for a few years. Just look. We'd be close to Savannah and Charleston, places we've always dreamed of visiting."

So, we did it.

We were still blazing our own trail. Arnie quit his job and covered home base again while I pursued a brand-new career. Our son Jonathan decided to come with us and enroll at Valencia Community College. Moving across the country would mean major changes for all of us, but the greater burden of getting us settled and anchored would fall on Arnie's shoulders.

During our first year, Arnie had done all the heavy lifting, finding new doctors, community resources, even grocery stores. When the first location ended up being too far for me to drive to work every day, he located an apartment for us just ten minutes from Disney.

Now I finally had the time and energy to look for nearby trails where I could get back to walking. Vicki Lavendol, a Disney colleague, told me about the West Orange Trail. "I'm not much of a walker, but I'd be happy to take you out there and go on a walk." We headed out. The trail was beautiful. I figured we could do a quick 10-mile walk like my good old Tucson days, but I was miserable after walking only five miles.

Somehow, I hadn't fully processed the fact that high humidity means there is so much moisture in the air that the sweat on your body doesn't evaporate. I no longer felt that amazingly fresh and invigorating sensation I had enjoyed in Arizona. The temperatures in Arizona could easily creep up to 100 degrees, but it was a *dry* heat. It evaporated. It cooled. It made me strong.

This wet heat made me weak. And old. *What have I done?*

I am usually pretty good at finding silver linings and there were many despite this oppressive humidity. Rachel was doing well in the Navy. Jonathan was getting settled in Valencia Community College. Arnie was taking a few classes too and was happily preparing to return to college full time for a Liberal Arts Master's Degree. I enjoyed working with other members of the organization development team, learning so much it almost felt like I was back in college. It was exhilarating.

But walking in this heat and humidity was debilitating. After one more mile I had to sit down on a rock by the trail to catch my breath. Vicki, who had said she was not much of a walker, was doing fine. She grew up in Florida.

I sat there taking a few miserable breaths, telling myself I had to get a grip. Then I started looking around at the spectacular green growth. Trees, flowers, bushes. It slowly dawned on me that flat damp Florida could also be beautiful.

"It's humidity, not a hurricane!" I quickly concluded. It would take some effort, but I knew I would not, *could* not let Florida weather dampen my spirit and zest for walking.

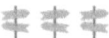

My mind snaps back to the marathon. We turn a corner and are marching down Magic Kingdom Main Street with cheering crowds lining both sides. Our marathon parade gets congested as walkers and runners are funneled into this narrow but lively space.

"Look, Kathy, we're keeping pace with some of the slower runners!" She gives me a thumbs-up as we wave, nod, and smile at all the happy guests.

We stride through a magical kaleidoscope of colors, smells, sounds. Buzz by food stalls and souvenir shops filled with pirate hats and swords. I pause for a moment in front of The Enchanted Tiki Room and remember my mom's glee when we took her to this same attraction at Disneyland in California as part of our 75th birthday gift to her. The spectacular multi-colored aviary show delighted her. Her smile was more brilliant than the birds.

We head through an open gate into the backstage area. Then glide by the half marathon finish line. I check my watch. It's 9:15. We have maintained a 13.5-minute per mile pace for the first half of the marathon!

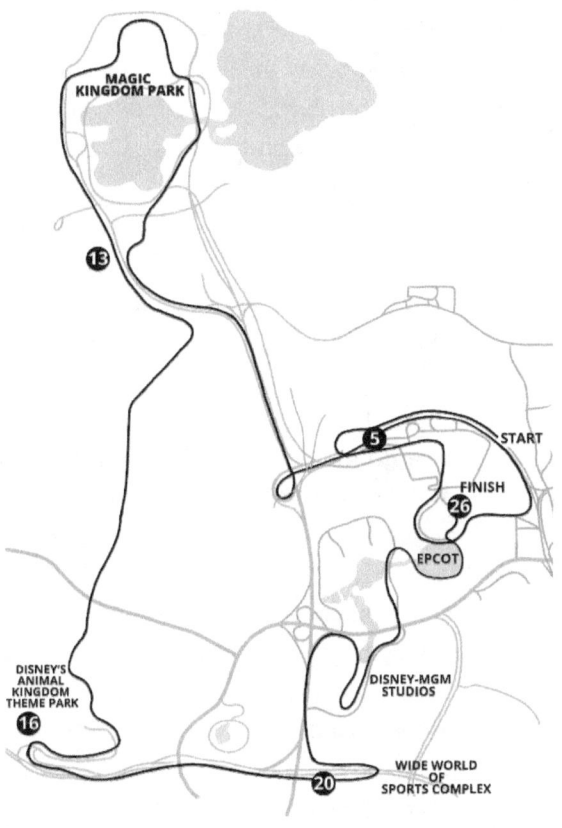

Soon, we find ourselves on a quiet, winding backroad that leads into Animal Kingdom. We pass through another backstage area filled with service trucks, equipment, and large grassy animal enclosures. We enter a lush green savanna accompanied by brief sounds of silence. Then step through one more gate. Suddenly we're back in the enthusiastic environment of another Main Street, this time with the Tree of Life on the left and Safari Village shops on the right. We become part of the entertainment again with guests waving and cheering us on.

We leave the park and pass Mile 16. Up to this point, our strength and spirits have been lifted by cool weather, attractions, and our new best friend, adrenaline. Going forward might not be quite as easy. "Kathy, I remember reading this road is long, straight, boring, and probably the toughest part of the route."

"Are we going to be okay?" Kathy looks worried. She has no sense of direction or distance and continues to rely heavily on me for progress reports and pep talks.

"We'll be fine," I promise her. "It's just not as entertaining and interesting as the first part. Our pace is a little slower but still good. We have four more miles to the final checkpoint at Mile 20. Then we'll spend most of the last six miles in and out of the other parks."

It's getting hot. There's no shade. We slow down a bit more. But then we hear a drumbeat and pick up our pace. The melody doesn't register but the beat lifts our spirits and our legs. We wave at the entertaining ensemble and keep walking, almost marching onward. The music fades.

Then we hear another beat in the distance. As we get closer, our pace picks up again as we stomp by a little group playing another bouncy tune. I start to laugh. "Leave it to Disney. As soon as the music from one band fades, we take a few steps in silence, and then another one picks up the rhythm. Keeping us entertained and motivated. Pretty darn cool."

We settle back into a comfortable stride, closer to a 16-minute-per-mile pace but still making good enough time. We are going to do it. I know it!

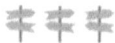

I let my mind wander back to that West Orange Trail trip. On the way home I kept trying to calm down. Cool down. Then I felt a little chill when I remembered that vacant lot next door. "Vicki, do you know what used to be in the lot by our apartment complex?"

Vicki nodded. "Oh, yes. That used to be a Jellystone Park campground. It was quite beautiful. They closed it a few years ago and made everyone move out because they were going to build another apartment complex, but it's just been sitting there."

When we moved to the apartment, I started walking along the busy street. It was loud with little natural beauty, lots of trash scattered along the sidewalk. I longed for the serenity of Sabino Canyon, my haven.

I had seen multiple signs with dire warnings of "Danger," "Construction Site," "No Trespassing," dangling on the chain link fence of this vacant lot. Pieces of rusted construction equipment were planted behind the fence. Behind that detritus was a large vacant lot with mounds of dirt. But surrounding that abandoned construction site was a majestic stand of tall trees and lush undergrowth. If I squinted my eyes and focused on the green circumference, it looked like a little nature preserve. I felt a refreshing wave of anticipation just thinking about that abandoned campground right next door.

It's 11:00 as we turn onto the road that leads to the Wide World of Sports parking lot and the Mile 20 checkpoint. We pause at the water stop and then loop back down the same road. There's Arnie! Standing over on the right, waving at us. "You both look great!" he says. "How do you feel?"

We both wave, delighted to see that beautiful familiar face in the crowd. "Fine! I've been tracking our pace, and we should complete right about the time I told you we would."

We cross the road heading up a small hill and look back on the last few miles of the long road from Animal Kingdom. One hundred or so walkers are still a few miles behind us. And just behind them are the cleaning crews. "I hope they make it. They're so close," Kathy says.

"They should be fine. It looks like we'll cross the finish line with a half hour to spare. If they make it to Mile 20, they will be allowed to finish even if it takes them longer than seven hours. From everything I read, they give everyone a chance if they're within the checkpoint guidelines."

The last six miles fly by with another Main Street strut, this time through the Disney MGM Studios. We wave. We smile. We could get used to this. There's Winnie the Pooh and Eeyore too. And even the Green Army Men! So many characters. So tempting to stop for a picture with at least one of them. Can't take time. Maybe next year.

We head back into Epcot. The ranks have thinned out and we're in the back of the pack with perhaps 15-20 others close behind. No more cheering crowds. We look less like marathoners and more like park guests rushing to meet friends for lunch.

We turn the corner at Mile 26 with just .2 miles left. See a balloon arch. Hear cheers from a surprisingly large crowd. We cross the finish line of our very first marathon, bend our knees and bow to receive a Mickey Mouse Medal.

"Guess what, Kathy? Our timing was practically perfect. We finished in six hours and 35 minutes! How's that for a consistent pace?"

Kathy grins. Gives me a thumbs up as we hobble back to the car, both suddenly famished and exhausted.

Our adrenaline boost is fading.

Kathy drives. "I have my stuff with me. Is it still okay for me to hang out at your place for the rest of the day like we planned?"

"Absolutely! Arnie already loaded *Chariots of Fire* in the DVD. We can eat, chill, snack, and then order pizza for this evening."

We come to a stop light.

Kathy turns and asks, "You were so confident right from the start. You are 55 and this was your first marathon. Why? How could you overcome your fear? Why weren't you terrified?"

"I've asked myself that same question. I think my Grand Canyon experience changed me for good. I knew what I wanted and needed to do back then. Now I have this surprising sense of excitement, curiosity, and perspective. What's the worst that could happen? We get a free ride back to the finish line? It looked like it would be an adventure. So why not?"

I smile.

So does Kathy. "Thanks for inviting and encouraging me. Maybe you helped me discover my own kind of Grand Canyon moment. I'm no longer afraid to walk a marathon."

I feel a shock of exhilaration course through my body. *I motivated someone. May have changed her life.* That felt even better than completing my first marathon!

The light turns green.

Once Arnie was sure we would make it (although he said he never had a single doubt) he had rushed home to hang a "Congratulations" banner in our living room and to put finishing touches on our marathoners' brunch of scrambled eggs, bagels, lox, orange juice, and coffee. The perfect repast. Arnie never does these events with me, but he is *always* by my side in my heart. He encourages me, uplifts me, and makes sure I properly and deliciously celebrate each event.

As I relax, I remember one more trip back to that lot next door.

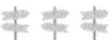

After my West Orange Trail meltdown with Vicki, I renewed my vow and refused to let Florida humidity dampen my spirit. I would and could stay happily active in a beautiful space. So, the next day after work I walked along the tall chain link fence that separated our apartment complex from the former Jellystone Campground. I inched around bushes that hid the bottom portion of the fence.

The fence was festooned with the same "Do Not Enter" and "No Trespassing - This Means You" signs that decorated the front. These signs were more than a little intimidating, especially since I'm usually a rule follower, but I kept advancing. Stepping. Looking. Sensing.

Then I saw it. A hole. Someone had already cut the fence and bent back the links to create a little crawl space. I gazed at that hole in the fence. Glanced at all the warning signs. Then looked around to see if anyone was watching. What the heck! I crawled through that hole in the fence, feeling a bit like Mary Lennox who found the key to the door that led to her *Secret Garden*.

Rocks littered the ground. It almost looked like a mountain trail. I was drawn in, unable to resist the magnetic pull of this green space. My heart was pounding. I saw a tiny path that had been created by someone stamping through the tallgrass. Others had come before me. I followed in their footsteps, walking slowly along the narrow, overgrown trail through a small stand of towering trees. The path curved behind all that old construction equipment in the front of the lot and ended up at a large mound of dirt. This little hill was not more than 15 feet high, but *any* elevation in Florida is a cause for celebration.

Then the trail continued around the mound like a little labyrinth gradually circling the pinnacle. Magical! I stood at the *peak* for a few minutes then hiked around and back down, tracing the trail on the side and to the back of the lot. I found another hill! Not as high, maybe 10 feet, but decidedly vertical.

I quickly mapped out a little trail. It looked like a giant "C" from the back hill winding along the side path through the trees, then over to the taller hill in front. I'd walk to the front hill, climb up and down two times, then follow the trail to the back hill, go up and down twice, then head back up to the front. It took me around 30 minutes to do three loops, about 2 miles.

I started crawling through the fence 3-4 times a week, walking, climbing my hills, feeling relaxed, peaceful, creative. My very own nature preserve.

In Arizona I usually hiked Sabino Canyon at least 2-3 times a week. It became my *regular* trail, providing the beauty, serenity, peace, and perspective I craved all year long. And now I found a new trail in Florida, right in my back yard! I could walk in my secret space as often as I wanted during the entire year.

My walking life was becoming comfortably balanced with shorter trails, longer training hikes, and occasional challenging, motivating events.

Later in 2000, Kathy answered a headhunter's call and accepted an executive-level job in another state. I started my own recruiting campaign to find a new walking partner for the WDW Marathon. I became not a headhunter, but a leg hunter.

I remembered that Vicki had gone on that first West Orange Trail hike with me last year. She could be a great marathon partner. But she had said she didn't consider herself much of a walker.

Start slow, Sandi. Be strategic. Help her discover the joy of walking and then suggest walking next year's marathon. I didn't want to scare her off.

When the summer heat retreated, Vicki was delighted to walk the West Orange Trail with me once a month. She was getting hooked. Even started coming over most Saturday mornings to walk 5 or 10 miles around our neighborhood. One time, we stretched our walk to 13 miles. (How strategic). It was time to make my pitch. "Vicki, we're having so much fun walking and talking together, how would you like to walk the Disney Marathon with me next year?"

She squinted. Gave me a look. Not a happy one. Started shaking her head. "Is that the one you and Kathy did last year? I don't know, Sandi. I'm tired after we walk 10 miles, I don't think

I could ever walk 26 miles."

"Well, consider this," I said as I moved in to close the deal. "We just walked 13 miles and if we can take a 13-mile walk every weekend for the next three months, we can easily complete the marathon." I thought that was a compelling argument. Vicki didn't. At first.

After walking for a few more minutes, her *are you crazy?* look faded. She slowly conceded. "I'm not an athlete and I can't believe I'm agreeing to this, but yes, I'll do it with you."

We trained. Got stronger. Completed the marathon. Enjoyed our time together. And have continued walking together through the years.

Later when Vicki had incorporated marathon walking and running into her life, she never failed to thank me for encouraging her to get started on this new journey.

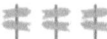

When I was young, I learned to look both ways before crossing the street. Now when I stand at a *life-change crosswalk* I have learned to scan the *entire* environment. To look, listen, feel. To notice little things—like the little yellow poster that invited me to attend an article-writing class. I responded and ended up writing a delightfully new and different chapter in my book of life.

At 55 I saw an email about the WDW Marathon. I signed up and added another satisfying dimension to my life. And even helped others do the same. Maybe I'll discover something new at 65 and even 75. Who knows what the future will hold?

What I *do* know is that I continue to reap significant benefits from scanning, paying attention, discovering, doing. Saying yes. A flyer. An email. A hole in the fence. So many options and opportunities to be noticed and embraced.

What else was out there waiting for me? I just needed to see it, seize it.

That answer came more quickly than I expected.

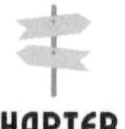

CHAPTER 4
Walking Together - Again

So, Sis, do you think I could walk the next Walt Disney World Marathon with you?" Chuck asked.

I was stunned. Delighted, but also hesitant. He was my big brother, older by two years, six foot five, former Green Beret. Looked like he had all the right stuff. But—this was a lot to absorb. How did we even get to this question?

I paused for a moment of gratitude. I had not even seen my brother in more than 20 years. And yet here we were walking and talking, just like when we were kids.

Chuck and his wife, Iva Jean, had come to Orlando for a visit. They wanted to get together with us and they really wanted to visit the Parks. So here we were, walking together on my little Jellystone Park trail.

"Your Mickey Mouse medals are awesome, and it sounds like you have had a great time walking through all the theme parks," Chuck said.

As we walked along, I remembered the joy we had shared when we grew up in Tucson, far away from our extended family back in Illinois. Mom made the most of what we had. And what we had were the mountains, deserts, canyons, and streams that surrounded Tucson. They became our playground. We were best buddies as we hiked, explored, climbed rocks, and splashed in mountain streams, especially in Sabino Canyon.

Then we grew up and went our separate ways after high

school. I went to one college. He went to another. I taught on the San Carlos Apache Reservation, got married, moved to New York for a year, then back to Arizona, and started working at the telephone company. Chuck joined the Army, got married, became a Green Beret, and flew a Huey medevac in Viet Nam.

I stayed in the Southwest. He settled in the Southeast. Even picked up a drawl. We were consumed with our own lives with no strong connection, especially after Mom died. We were not necessarily estranged. Just no compelling reason to be engaged. Not much in common anymore except our childhood memories.

When he popped the question about walking the next marathon with me, I should have been overjoyed. This could be a wonderful opportunity to do something together, to reconnect, to capture a bit of our childhood camaraderie. I just wasn't sure walking a marathon would be the best way for us to rekindle our relationship after all these years. I worried that my Mikey Mouse medal might be more appealing to him than walking the entire 26.2 miles to earn it.

And I'm a bit of a control freak. Walking with Chuck would be way different than walking with Kathy or Vicki. I would lose that control with my brother, especially since we would be training in separate states. Plus—he *was* my older brother.

I reminded myself that jumping into unknown territory is good. Even life changing.

So, I said yes. Then immediately peppered him with questions and expectations, truly living up to my role as the bossy baby sister. "Are you sure you can train enough? Vicki and I have already started walking and training for next year. Do you have good shoes? You can't just stroll. You must push your pace at least a few times each month."

He nodded emphatically. "I've been riding my bike to work, but I can start walking at least a few days a week. And I'll buy better shoes."

"Do you promise?" I persisted, "I know how much you hate

to buy expensive shoes. If you buy good shoes, then I'll pay for your registration and get us registered for next year. Deal?"

"Deal!"

Our plans were put to a test during that summer when Kathy, my first marathon buddy, called me with big news. "Sandi, I just got a call from a headhunter recruiting someone with a PhD and organization development experience for an OD Director job at Limited Brands in Columbus, Ohio. I'm happy where I am and am not ready to move, so can I give her your name?"

The timing was perfect. I had worked at Disney for three years and the company had just initiated a voluntary down-sizing initiative to cut costs. "Sure," I said. "This might be the perfect time to make a move."

The headhunter called the next day. We video conferenced a few days later. She liked what she heard and saw. Arnie and I started a whirlwind of trips to Columbus. Limited Brands was interested in enticing spouses as well as recruiting candidates, so while a real estate agent drove Arnie around the city, I went through several rounds of interviews.

When I received the job offer, I had one additional request. "My husband has one semester left in his master's degree program at Rollins. Is it possible to expand my hiring bonus to cover expenses for him to fly back and forth to Orlando so he can complete his program?" And in line with Limited Brands' dual focus on employees and their spouses, the extra funds were approved. We were on our way.

We had to pack, find temporary housing, and help Jonathan figure out where he would live since he wanted to stay in Orlando.

And I had to call my brother.

"Chuck, we're moving to Columbus, Ohio for a new job, but I'd be happy to fly back to Orlando next January to do the marathon with you if you still want to do it. Jonathan is staying here so we can bunk with him."

"Absolutely! I can't wait to get one of those Mickey Mouse

medals!"

"Okay," I said. "Are you still training?"

"I am, and I got some new shoes too."

"Okay! We can still make this work."

And we did. Sort of. I kept in touch with Vicki. We both felt confident our separate training activities were just what we needed for another successful walk through the Parks. Chuck drove to Orlando. I flew. We picked up our goodie bags at the Expo and were ready to go. Or so I thought.

As we surveyed our stuff in Jonathan's apartment the night before, I noticed Chuck's backpack stuffed full of supplies. "You don't need all that food, Chuck. They have water and snacks on the route. That extra weight could slow you down, make it harder to keep on pace."

He set his jaw. "This is what I carry when I walk, and I need a couple bottles of my quinine water."

I looked at his shoes. Blinked. "Chuck, those are old Walmart shoes. I thought you were going to get fitted and buy good walking shoes."

"These were the most expensive ones I could find at Walmart!" he said. "The clerk said they looked fine on my feet, and they would be perfect for a long walk. I've been wearing them for the past year during all my walks. They got wet a few times, but they feel fine."

Then I saw a brand-new navy-blue Champion sweatshirt. There was no way he would want to toss that. "It's cold when we start, but it gets pretty hot during the last part of the race. I'm afraid you're going to get overheated."

Chuck had his plan, and he was sticking to it. "If I get too hot, I can take it off and put it in my backpack. I want to keep it."

I needed to back off. "Okay, just remember, we have to keep a steady fast pace so we don't get swept."

"Sis, I've trained. I know best what I need."

I started to say, "You don't know how to walk a marathon,"

but I bit my tongue.

He continued, "I can do this with absolutely no problem."

There were problems.

Our start was good. Vicki and I walked on either side of Chuck, pointing out the Walt Disney World landmarks, chatting about some of the fun things we got to do as Cast Members. Time flew by. I monitored Chuck at each water station, making sure he was drinking. He noticed I was watching and lifted his big bottle of quinine. "I'm drinking this. I'm fine!"

We made good time around and out of Epcot, through Magic Kingdom, the half marathon checkpoint, and even Animal Kingdom. But it was getting warmer on that long straight road to the Wide World of Sports complex. Chuck slowed down. He looked damp and depleted. "It's pretty hot, Chuck," I said. "Do you want to take off your sweatshirt?"

"No."

"Are you drinking and eating enough?"

"Yes!"

At Mile 18 Chuck was limping on his worn-out shoes. Walking slower. I walked in front of him trying to set the pace. That worked for about a mile. Then he started lagging further behind, so I stepped back to walk beside him.

"Are you okay?" I asked. "Do you want to eat something from your pack? I have some M&M's. Do you want them?" Chuck kept walking slowly, looking down, and shook his head. "Please drink some more of your water, okay?" He did.

Finally, we passed Mile 20 and did not have to worry about getting swept. But I was starting to wonder if he would even make it to the finish line. It was clear he required more than reminders and offers. I needed to get his attention.

"Chuck, we have six more miles to go and I'm not sure we're going to make it."

Chuck stopped, stunned. Reality registered. He might not get his medal? This was getting serious. "Okay. What do I need to do?"

I issued a cadence of commands in military style: (Chuck could relate to that.)

> Take off your sweatshirt.
> Drink the rest of the quinine in your bottle.
> Put your sweatshirt in your backpack.
> Give your backpack to me.
> Walk between me and Vicki.
> Put your hands on our shoulders.
> Now!

Chuck obeyed. The path was wide enough so we could walk together for the final six miles at a slow but steady pace. I imagine we were quite the sight with 5'2" Vicki on the left, 5'10" me on the right, and 6'5" Chuck in the middle leaning on us. But at this point, lots of people were hobbling, struggling, doing whatever was needed to get to the finish line.

We stopped at the final water station. The volunteers saw our looks and offered empathetic encouragement along with cups of water. "Keep going! You are so close. You got this!"

I made sure Chuck was drinking and eating but wasn't sure if he was getting enough fuel to catch up. I couldn't keep nagging him, so I just kept patting his hand on my shoulder, hoping he had enough strength to make it to the end.

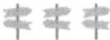

The pictures from the marathon show the three of us crossing the finish line, smiling, holding our hands up high. Our time was 7:05, slightly over the seven-hour time limit but fine since we had passed Mile 20 in time. Even at our slow pace there were more than 70 walkers behind us who still crossed the finish line without getting swept.

Chuck bowed to receive his Mickey Mouse medal. "Thank you, Sis!"

Then he leaned his back against a makeshift wall and slid down to a sitting position murmuring, "I don't feel so good." Vicki and I propped him up and helped him limp over to the medical tent. The medics hauled him to a cot.

"He looks pretty dazed, almost like it's dementia," one doctor said.

"What the heck!" I thought. "He's only 59!"

"He's totally depleted. Let's get him started on an IV." After about a half-hour, they transported him to Sand Lake Hospital to get him stabilized. Vicki and I went to the emergency room to wait. Two hours later, he walked into the waiting room on the arm of a medical assistant. He looked a little weak and sheepish. He nodded and gave a wan smile. "Thank you both."

By the next morning he seemed fine as we headed back to the Expo to shop and pick up our finisher's certificates. Chuck bought a marathon sweatshirt and Mickey Mouse hat to go along with his Mickey Mouse marathon medal.

And with a big smile he said, "So Sis, do you think we can we do this again next year?"

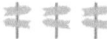

It was a rocky start for me and Chuck. Here we were walking a marathon together after years of living our lives on opposite sides of the country, in different communities, and sometimes on what seemed like separate planets. We walked those first 26.2 miles together playing a typical brother-sister back and forth between my demands and Chuck's needs.

But it still felt good. We wanted to make it work. We moved forward and pulled together in a way that surprised and delighted both of us.

That first marathon with Chuck provided valuable life

lessons as most challenging new situations usually do. Participating in events with family and friends can get tricky and sticky. They can also be incredibly renewing and rewarding, even transformative.

Chuck and I created an entirely new relationship. He adjusted. I relaxed. We discovered a new middle ground.

And we returned to walk another WDW Marathon the following January.

We finished our second marathon together in 6 hours and 46 minutes. He felt fine. I felt fine. We did great.

Chuck took me to the airport to drop me off before he drove home to Virginia. We hugged goodbye. Then he broke down. Through his tears he said, "I'm so glad we can do these marathons together. It means more to me than you'll ever know. Thank you. Love you."

We headed out, each of us believing we would return and repeat our adventure the following year.

But we never made it back to Orlando and never again walked a full marathon together.

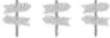

By the following year, I was struggling with my degenerating right hip. Chuck was due for his first spinal surgery.

We put our marathons on hold for a few years, but we missed them and missed each other. In 2007, after both of us had healed from our first round of surgeries, we started walking half marathons together in Columbus, Ohio. Chuck drove from his home in Virginia.

We walked three half marathons before Chuck was diagnosed with multiple myeloma and became too weak to walk long distances. Even 5Ks were no longer an option.

Our walking days had ended, but we still had our medals and photographs. We had our stories. Those fun, hilarious, and heartwarming walking sagas. Just five events. A new lifetime of precious memories.

Thank goodness we started our marathon journey when we did, before it was too late. Thank goodness we took advantage of that brief window in time.

Chuck and I did not give up on each other. We did not quit. We made it work. We mellowed and merged into a new and rewarding relationship that endures to this day.

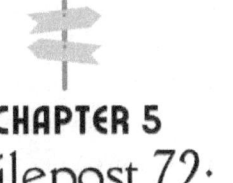

CHAPTER 5
Milepost 72:
Answering the Call
of the Inca Trail

"I'm not sure I can do this!"

I had been retired for almost two years, but I still hadn't taken a big trip. Was I scared? Getting too comfortable? Too set in my ways? Was I worried about leaving Arnie alone? What was going on?

Then one day Arnie walked into my office, something obviously weighing on his mind. He had already declared he was done with flying, especially long distances, but he had consistently urged me to pursue my travel dreams. "Sandi, we are making the most of our time together, but you haven't taken any trips yet. I told you not to hold back because of me. I want you to take trips, little ones, especially big ones. It's what you have always wanted. It's what I want for you. I just don't want you to resent me for not going with you."

I blinked. Surprised. "Of course, not. I'm not sure why I haven't headed off yet. It just seemed like we were finally getting settled. Maybe I didn't want to jeopardize that serenity. And maybe, even though you have always encouraged me, I didn't want you to resent me for leaving you alone."

Now Arnie blinked. "Of course, not. You need to get going. I won't be totally alone, and I'll be with you in spirit all the way."

Then, as if I needed even more encouragement, during a trip

to Maryland, as Rachel and I watched a TV segment on Machu Picchu, she asked, "Mom, when are you going to start taking some of those big trips you always talked about doing after you retired? You wanted me and Jonathan to go with you on some trips since Dad doesn't like big trips. So how about Peru?"

I agreed. "It's time to get going."

Jonathan could not leave his U.S. Navy assignment, so Rachel and I just did it. I used my passport for the first time. That was a big step.

My first trip out of North America was everything I could have imagined and more. And something happened on that first trip that demanded we return to Peru the following year.

We had climbed up to Sun Gate (*Intipunku* in Quechua) at Machu Picchu. At first, our eyes were riveted on the verdant terraces and ancient stone ruins far below. But then we turned left and saw a woman and her guide hiking up a steep rocky trail. It called my name.

"Rachel, we have to come back next year and hike the Inca Trail."

I quickly learned that hearing a call is one thing. Making it happen is another.

We started planning for our 2016 Inca Trail Trek soon after we returned. We were also training for a Grand Canyon rim-to-rim (R2R) in October.

Then we hit a few snags. More than a few.

When our first travel agent was not able to secure a spot for us with a tour company for the Inca Trail Trek, she said it was too late. We put our plans on the back burner, figuring we'd have to wait another year.

Then I ended up getting tendonitis from overtraining, so Rachel and I cancelled our R2R. I decided to spend a week alone at the Grand Canyon, renewing my spirit, nursing my foot, and trying to convince myself not to give up.

After my canyon sojourn, I took a shuttle back to Flagstaff

where I would transfer to another shuttle to Phoenix. A young woman sitting behind me in the van was showing someone pictures of her recent Inca Trail Trek.

I whirled around in my seat. "Inca Trail? You just hiked the Inca Trail? My daughter and I wanted to go next year, but our plans fell through. The timing isn't right, and now I'm wondering whether I can even do it."

"Well, of course you can!" she said with astonishing authority. "I heard you telling the driver about hiking the Grand Canyon. If you can hike there, you can hike the Inca Trail. There are many reliable trekking companies that still have slots available for next year. I'm not in the best shape, but I did it. Of course, it was hard in some spots. And it was absolutely one of the biggest gifts I have ever given myself. Do *not* give up on your dream! Give me your contact information and I'll send you all my information," she commanded. (Interesting how some strangers can be so benevolently bossy.) I obeyed. She delivered.

I frequently encounter angels on a trail without learning their name or ever seeing them again. I met Ann Fazzini in a van. She got me right back on track, and we have stayed in contact through the years.

We found a new travel agent, Douglas, who secured a spot for us on a trek that was just a little later and possibly a bit hotter in July, but we were willing to take the chance. The great news was that our trek was back on track for next year.

But then I started a six-month battle with bursitis that was soon joined with sciatica pain. The stabbing ricocheting pain that traveled up and down my left leg was so excruciating I could barely walk and even had trouble sleeping.

I refused to give up. I kept walking, slowly nursing the pain. Finally, after PT visits, home exercises, and three spinal injections, my nerve pain calmed down.

And then just four months before our trek, Arnie and I were walking slowly to the mailbox when I felt and even heard a snap in my right foot. "Ouch!"

"What's the matter?" Arnie asked.

"Something happened in my foot. It feels like something broke, but that doesn't make sense." We continued our walk home. By the time we arrived, my right foot was red and swollen.

I was able to get an appointment the next week. The X-ray showed a break right in the middle of my foot. It was March. I told the orthopedist about the Inca Trail Trek we had scheduled for July.

"So, what happens now?" I asked.

"Well, not much," he responded. "It's a clean break, not too jagged, so there's no point in a cast. I'm not going to boot you. You're an athlete. You know the drill. Rest as much as you can for the next few weeks, then walk slowly for shorter distances, stopping if it hurts or starts swelling, and then gradually build your distance and strength back up. Just don't overdo it."

I appreciated that he saw an "athlete" in me—right along with my wrinkles, gray hair, and broken foot. I followed his instructions. My foot slowly healed.

I refused to consider these aches and breaks as a sign I should give up my quest.

Finally, in July, we made it back to Peru.

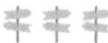

It was the *dreaded* Day 2 of our 4-day 3-night Inca Trail Trek, 4:30 a.m., and chilly high in the Andes. We were nestled in a blue tent our porters had pitched on a rocky patch of green surrounded by trees, setting us slightly apart from the other campsites.

A porter "knocked" on our tent door, "Good morning! Warm water here." I'd been awake, snuggled deep in my sleeping bag for some time thinking back to the online descriptions of this day. At first, these tales terrified and almost convinced me I couldn't do it, even after Ann had insisted I could. Almost every story was written by people much younger than me. Not one of the posts ever referred to this as simply "Day 2." It was always accompanied with words such as *ominous, knee busting, infamous, bloody hard.* It was unanimous. Day 2 would earn all those dire adjectives because we would hike up to the 14K summit of Dead Woman's Pass. It was a small comfort to know that while the pass when viewed from the back side looks like a dead woman lying on her back, it was *not* named for some woman who actually died there.

But as I read, I noticed every one of these stories ended in success. Even though they were filled with words like *exhausted, crying, sobbing, hobbling, unrelenting pain, overwhelming fatigue, incredibly slow*—every trekker made it!

These posts also included helpful tips that had helped these intrepid explorers reach the summit and achieve their dream. On our first trip to Peru, Rachel and I had already picked up a few tips of our own. Especially the value of coca leaf used to reduce the effects of elevation sickness in the Andes. We had even acquired a taste for the slightly-bitter, strongly-healing tea. Yes, these leaves are a source of cocaine. We can't take any home with us. But here in Peru, it's our legal drug of choice. A mild stimulant that is a helpful *altitude* aid and *attitude* pick up.

We also knew we were in good hands since our competent travel agent Douglas had selected a tour company that was reliable and treated its porters well. I'll never forget his response when I asked if it made sense to pay for an extra porter even though it would just be the two of us. "It's well worth the extra $150. It makes things a little easier on the other porters, you get a private bathroom tent, and you're providing much-needed employment with a reputable company."

I had slept just a few hours because my right foot started to twitch every 2-3 minutes, preventing me from getting into a deep sleep, which meant my bladder did not have to work too hard to get my attention. I crawled out of my sleeping bag, trying not to wake Rachel, slipped on my shoes, and padded over to our bathroom tent. After my 10th trip, I was exhausted and frustrated. But even then, I couldn't help but notice the starry night sky high in the Andes. In this luminescent aura and spirit of gratitude and appreciation, I decided to refer to the more lyrical Inca name of *Warmiwanusca* for the 14K summit of today's trek.

Rachel and I shimmied out of our bags and got ready for the day. This was our first morning on the trek, yet we moved like veterans: quick, efficient, determined to be on time, even early. We're both hard-core rule followers. And it helped that Rachel by this time actually was a veteran and had served in the U.S. Navy for seven years. She knew how to pack small and manage quickly and efficiently in tiny berths on aircraft carriers and in barracks.

Breakfast was scheduled for 5:30. We climbed out of our tent, made a quick trip to our bathroom tent, and sat on our little folding chairs at the small table covered with a colorful cloth in the meal tent by 5:15. Miguel, our chef, had prepared a hearty meal of eggs, bacon, and breads. Jesus, one of the porters, started serving us as soon as we sat down. Frank joined us a few minutes later, surprised we were already eating. "Thank you! Not many trekkers in my previous tours have been so prompt and serious about getting an early start."

Frank, 5'5, slender, with a big-smile, and quite cute, had already served as our guide for our two days of easy, acclimating excursions before starting our Inca Trail Trek. At 31, he was nine years younger than Rachel's 40 years and less than half of my 72 years. He had grown up in Cusco, and was fluent in Spanish, English, and Quechua, the Indigenous language spoken by many locals in the Andes. He had earned a trove of formal tour-guide certificates, but it was his passion for noticing, capturing, and being captivated by natural beauty that truly set him apart.

When we told him we had already seen several churches during our first trip to Peru, he said, "So, how about this? Do you trust me to take you some place special that I can't tell you about right now?"

Later he took us to Oropesa, considered the Bread Capital of Peru, to a little neighborhood bakery to witness the making of *pan chuta,* a large disk-shaped bread with a sweet anise flavor. We were greeted and waved into a back room so we could watch the mixing process. Frank didn't even need to translate because the three women's expressions and gestures told us everything we needed to know. We moved to the front room to watch two young men placing loaves into the flaming opening of a small stone oven filled with eucalyptus leaves. We walked to a front yard ramada to see dozens of loaves resting on cooling racks. Frank bought two loaves—one for him and one for us. As Frank drove us back to Cusco, we all munched on that warm uniquely-tasty bread. No butter or jam needed. Unforgettable.

Our next experience was not as tasty. Yesterday, Frank had taught us how to take a small bunch of 4-5 dried coca leaves, stuff them in our cheek to soak them with our saliva, chew the wad like gum until it lost its taste, then deposit it in a tissue and start all over again. Who knows? At some point, we may even start to like that bitter, slimy blob. We already appreciated its effects.

We ate as much breakfast as we could, treating food as fuel, knowing we would need every calorie for today's trek. Then we grabbed our backpacks and my hiking poles from the tent, filled our water bottles, and met up with Frank who flashed another big smile. "I thought we would head out by 7:00, and here we are all ready by 6:00," he said. "Let's hit the trail. It will be a long day." I could see in his eyes he was worried, especially after I told him I didn't get much sleep last night. He told me yesterday I was one of the oldest women he has guided on this trek. Men, yes. Women, no. I did fine on our first day. He knew I was strong but slow. How I will handle this daunting climb is still unknown to him. At this point I knew I'd make it. I was a bit frustrated he was acting concerned. But that was his job. And he didn't know me.

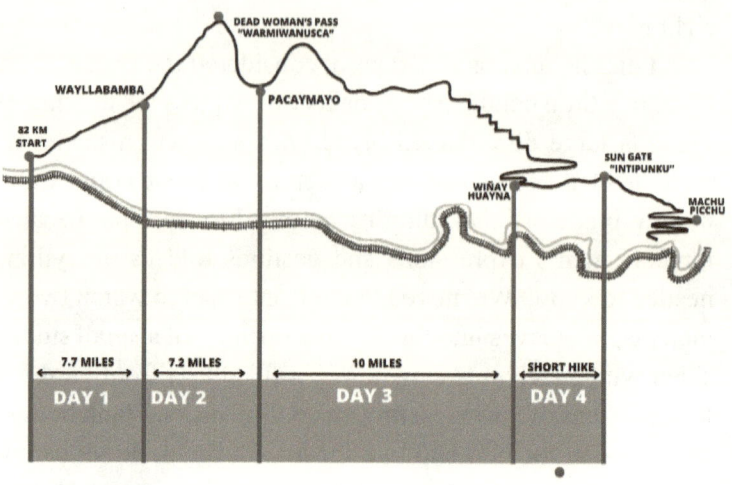

We headed out and gleefully noticed all the bugs that had plagued us yesterday when we started our hike at the lower elevation had disappeared. This first portion was uphill but not as steep as what loomed ahead. We climbed step by step, a walking meditation through cloud forests with boughed branches, birds singing, beauty all around. Frank paused to describe and name orchids, hummingbirds, and unusually intriguing trees.

What a pleasant surprise! I knew we would be more comfortable hiking alone rather than in a big group, but I never expected this up-close-and-personal on-going education as we hiked.

Although we couldn't ignore the weight of what was coming ahead, it was clear Frank didn't want us to miss the joy of the journey. We walked over a tiny antique bridge of small branches tethered together as Frank carefully pointed out its unique construction. Because we had started an hour early, we were still ahead most others at Wayllabamba, last night's camp site.

At 9:30 we burst into the bright sun at the Lepaca rest stop. This broad flat saddle area is the final staging area before the assent up Dead Woman's Pass. "We will rest here for about 30 minutes," Frank said as he poured us each a cup of coca tea from his thermos. "Please start chewing some leaves. It will be a big help with this altitude. I will contact our porters to let them know where we are." Our porters had already run ahead carrying their 45-pound packs filled with the tents, food, and other supplies needed to support our trek.

I sat on a log gazing at the amazing sights, feeling like I was in a National Geographic documentary, perched at the treeline in the Andes. Other hikers and porters sped by, heading up the trail. Rachel walked over to a set of tables covered with multi-colored woven cloths. This little pop-up vending site was the final spot to buy snacks. People from local villages trek up here each day to sell an array of goodies providing nutrition for hikers and a source of income for them.

Rachel walked back from the snack table with a big smile and a little can of Pringles. "Here's something shiny to entice you to eat a little more." We both grinned as we remembered our walks with the shiny dimes I had tossed those many years ago. Our roles were shifting with her becoming more of the caretaker, and unfortunately, the greater worrier.

"Hon, I'll be fine. I can do this." We looked up at the final portion, a long winding trail carved into the mountain. Lots of rocks and places to huddle in the shade on the mountain side. A gradual drop-off with fascinating bushes, grasses, and flowers on the other side. I gave Rachel a big smile, grabbed my hiking poles, and we were off.

I was a little tired, a tiny bit scared, but adrenaline and coca tea were kicking in. I would do this. I'd be slow, but I'd make it to the top. I started chewing a few more coca leaves just to be sure.

Frank walked just ahead of me, pointing out steps with quiet guidance. "Walk back and forth, back and forth. We don't walk straight up. We weave back and forth across the trail like tiny switchbacks. It takes a few more steps but is much easier on your body. Back and forth, back and forth."

We slowly climbed as a meditative aura infused the

atmosphere. I fell into a state of mindfulness (or maybe a coca-leaf induced trance), paying attention, step by step. First was a soft symphony of footsteps, pole strikes, and Frank's soft crooning, *back and forth, back and forth.* Then the cymbal crash of chatter and cheers from groups ahead and behind as we leap-frogged up the trail.

Then Frank switched to a soft song. "Step here, step there," joined by Rachel, "Are you doing okay, Mom?" and finally I joined in, "Thanks, hon, I'm fine. How about you?" She responded, "I'm fine." Then the song repeated. "Step here, step there, back and forth, back and forth…"

I climbed 100 steps, stopped, and breathed deep. I saw the sunlit sky surrounded by the spectacular beauty of surrounding mountains, slow moving clouds, soft waving saw grass. The sidewinding snake dance continued, slowly ascending to the saddle of *Warmiwanusca.* Soft switchbacks made the steep climb possible. "Step here, step there. Back and forth, back and forth."

The music stopped abruptly as we looked ahead and saw two young women sick and sobbing, huddled by the trail. They were strangers, but that didn't matter to Frank. He was a trail guide for all on this trail. The women were dressed in dark clothes with no head covering, overheated, and dehydrated. "Just keep going up, remember to weave. I'll catch up with you," said Frank as he stopped to help them. He carried extra supplies, gave them water to drink, and started sprinkling water on their scarves and heads.

I hated seeing those women struggle and was grateful Frank could help them.

We kept moving forward on our own. "Look, Rachel!" I exclaimed as I pointed to a llama on the side of the trail.

"Yes! I got a great picture of it," said Rachel. "I'm taking as many as I can. It's so beautiful." She paused. "Are you doing okay, Mom?"

"Thanks, hon, I'm fine. How about you?" I turned and noticed Rachel was smiling, relaxing a bit, her worried look fading. *Oh good. Maybe she's catching my confidence.*

"I'm fine."

I stopped to sit on a nice flat rock right by the path, drank some water, breathed the crisp air that was almost electric. We continued climbing. Soon Frank rejoined us with an update. "They'll be okay. Just need some time to hydrate and huddle in the shade."

We could see 10-15 people at the top, waving and cheering other members of their group who were in front and behind us. It was crowded as we took turns stepping to the side of the trail that had narrowed to about 5 feet, letting small groups of people pass, then passing them as they paused to breathe.

The final 80-100 steps were the steepest of all. I remembered reading and dreaming about this. Visualization is a wonderful thing. I was prepared. *Breathe in through nose; breathe out through mouth.* Step 1, 2, 3, 4, 5. Pause. Step again. And up, up, up.

At 12:40, we made it to the top. I turned to smile at Rachel. She was crying. I started to cry too. We sat together on a rock at the 14K foot summit of Dead Woman's Pass on the Inca Trail, holding hands, trying to catch our breath. Not because it was hard to breathe in that rarified air, but because we were overwhelmed with joy. I dried my tears. Rachel was still crying.

"Mom, I knew how much you wanted this. I was worried even though you trained so hard and never gave up. I just wanted this so badly for you. For us." She sniffled. "All those people started cheering when you got to the top, and I wanted to shout out, 'You have no idea how strong my mom is! She is 72 years old with artificial hips and knees, atrial fib, and a not-quite-healed broken foot. And she did it! My mom just hiked up Dead Woman's Pass and she was not even the last person up!'"

We were happy. We were relieved. We were lucky. The weather had cooperated with brilliant clear blue skies. The sun that was blindingly hot when we first left the treeline at Lepaca now provided a warm embrace as we sat resting, daring to celebrate. I thought I heard Leonard Cohen singing "Hallelujah" somewhere in the background. But then maybe not.

We couldn't spend much more time in this high altitude. Even in the sun we started to get chilly. But we needed just a few more minutes to bask in our gratitude and wonder, and to remember how this journey began.

"Rachel, this never would have happened if we hadn't hiked up to Sun Gate when we visited Machu Picchu during our first Peru trip last year. If we hadn't hiked up, we would have never seen the Inca Trail. If we had not paused and looked down on that trail, I would never have heard that call or felt that pull. Even now I can feel that fierce force clutching my chest when we watched that woman hike slowly up the steps with her guide. This is a journey most people will never take. But we did. We are so fortunate."

Rachel stopped crying. "I wanted this for you so bad it hurt in my heart and my head." Frank started rubbing some oil on Rachel's neck and massaging the back of her head trying to soothe her raging headache, probably caused more by stress and concern for me than the altitude.

"I think there's a strong possibility that if we hadn't hiked the Grand Canyon all those years ago, we may not have even considered this. Do you think this was as hard as that was?" I asked.

"No," said Rachel. "The rim-to-rim-to-rim was harder because it was our first *ultra*. Even though we had trained we really didn't know what to expect. We've come a long, long way since the Grand Canyon. This is just another step on that journey we started way back then."

We took a few more photos. And then we posed for that iconic "We did it!" photo by the Warmiwanusca 4,215 m post. No more tears. Just smiles.

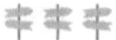

On Day 4, our last day, we sat on the wall with Frank as he pointed out constellations, enjoying the serenity of the early morning sky. Suddenly we heard a stampede of other hikers heading out for the final portion of the hike. Their pressing goal was to reach Sun Gate at Machu Picchu right before sunrise. I had read stories about this mad dash, how hikers had been injured as they trampled and crowded together on the narrow rocky trail.

We were delighted to stay out of the fray as we sat and star gazed. Later when the trail cleared, we walked in peace, listening to birdsong and feeling our elation and the elevation rise as we neared the end. We passed by deep mountain valleys and more ancient ruins. We stopped to investigate tiny flowers, plaques, and markers along the way.

On one final set of narrow steep stairs, Frank directed me to give my poles to Rachel and climb up using my hands and feet. I felt safe and secure as I motored up the trail on all fours.

Then we stopped. That final rocky portion of the Inca Trail loomed ahead. This was the section we saw a year ago when we gazed down from Sun Gate. Rachel and I looked at each other. "Mom, you take the lead."

I struggled to catch my breath, calm my heart, and squint the burn from my eyes. Then I took my first step. Our final journey felt spiritual. This time there was no doubt. Leonard Cohen *was* singing "Hallelujah" as we hiked up those ancient stone steps. One year ago, this trail had called to me. We had answered the call.

It was blissfully quiet when we stepped up onto Sun Gate. A solitary person stood over to the side. We missed the sunrise but arrived just as the sun aligned itself in a perfect position to shimmer through the majestic stone pillars. Beautiful and serene. Peaceful and calm. Our perfect ending.

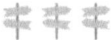

We revisited a few of our favorite spots in Machu Picchu,

surprised at how the crowds had increased in just one year. There were more restrictions, fewer opportunities to get close and feel the warmth emanating from the stones, structures, and shrines. Thank goodness we had not delayed this trip.

As we walked out the main entrance, I paused to embrace this moment as my heart and lungs filled with joy and gratitude. Then we waved goodbye to this beautiful, terraced citadel and took the bus down the mountain to Aguas Calientes, the little town known for its thermal baths that served as the gateway to Machu Picchu.

Frank wanted to escort us to our hotel before he took the train back to Cusco. We said our goodbyes as we huddled around a little table in a lush green garden at our hotel, sitting, drinking tea, reminiscing, sharing appreciation. We even "friended" each other on Facebook.

The Inca Trail portion of our journey had come to an end. Tomorrow we would hop on the train back to Cusco. And the next day enjoy a multi-stop bus trip down to Punto to tour Lake Titicaca. But for today, Rachel and I would bathe and bask in the first shower we had taken in four days. Then fully refreshed, we would return to the garden to sit surrounded by the beautiful foliage and bountiful memories of our great adventure. And celebrate another life-changing experience.

Later back home, as I reflected on my emerging 70s, I had no idea retirement could open so many doors. Be so satisfying. Savoring sweet moments at home with Arnie. Traveling at home and abroad. I looked ahead with anticipation, curiosity, and a sense of urgency, determined to embrace the unknown, listen to other calls, and answer them.

Who would join me? Where would we go? What new opportunities were waiting?

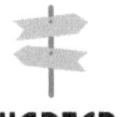

CHAPTER 6
Milepost 73:
Embracing Balance in China

Since I retired, not one trip had been perfect. Each had some element of risk or level of inconvenience. I hadn't realized that my resilience muscles would be strengthened by embracing new challenges and overcoming setbacks. I figured I'd learn more, do more, and see more. But I never expected to *become* more.

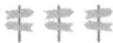

"Jonathan would love this!" emailed Rachel. She knew I had wanted to take her younger brother on a big trip since he had not been able to go with us to Peru, so she sent me an ad for a *Great Wall Marathon*.

"I didn't have any big trips planned for 2017. This just might work out. Thanks, hon. Jonathan wanted to have a new goal after completing the Ironman and moving here last year. This trip isn't scheduled until May, so he'd have lots of time to train."

"And this time maybe you can even include your grandson," said Rachel. "He also told me Flip wants to see China. This event includes a half marathon and 8.5K options. Maybe you two could do the fun run while Jonathan runs the marathon. It's a quick trip, just a week. You wouldn't be able to see and do the whole China thing while you're there, but it looks like a perfect opportunity for the three of you."

Jonathan loved the idea, especially since it was just a week, so he would not use too much leave and Flip would not miss too much school.

When Jonathan and the boys came down for the weekend, he and I ambled down to the Intracoastal Waterway trail for our usual 5k. We started our walk talking about our China adventure.

Then Jonathan's pace slowed. "Mom, you and Dad have helped me and Rachel financially and now, you're going to pay for this China trip. I know you two are doing fine, but I worry about your finances. You still tip big and make even bigger donations. But what if something happens? Will you be okay? Rachel and I would always take care of you, but I just don't want you to struggle."

I responded, "You know we made the choice to spend more money during the early years of our retirement through our 70s. I'm not being morbid, but I feel a certain sense of urgency. Who knows what will happen to us or the world in a few years? You and Rachel already know we are spending your inheritance now."

He nodded, "I know, but look at all the people who have lost their savings."

I tried again. "If our only priority was security, you'd be right: it would be easier to simply save as much as we can right now in case something happens. But we would do that out of fear. It would not be nearly so rewarding."

We continued walking. "Remember, hon, Dad and I both grew up with single moms. In the 50s, our families were called *broken*. Sometimes we were broke, but never broken. We lived small. When Chuck and I were growing up, we moved from one rental to another eleven times in eight years. Grandma kept finding slightly better places, one move at a time. At one point we lived in a Wingfoot house that was less than 250 square feet. It must have been hard on her, but to me and Chuck, our lives seemed perfectly normal."

"What's a Wingfoot?"

"Why don't you google it," I said. "My point is, even if all our savings were wiped out, we still have that tiny cabin in Maryland we bought 10 years ago. Dad and I wanted a home base where we could gather for family celebrations. If the bottom dropped out of everything, we could move to that cabin and live on our Social Security. That's an *incredible* worst-case scenario. This is how we want to live our lives."

We walked. Jonathan processed.

"Okie, dokie. A three-generation trip to China. Nice! Thank you!" Jonathan laughed. We walked back home, stepping a little lighter than when we started out.

Later in the day, our youngest grandson, seven-year-old Sam, and I walked down the street to our mailbox. Actually, I walked. Sam, the *treasure seeker*, bounced from one side of the road to the other, sort of like Tigger, picking up pinecones, acorns, and other fascinating items. Last year when we walked the Turtle Trot 5K along Fernandina Beach at Amelia Island, Jonathan and Flip ran ahead. Sam stayed with me crisscrossing from shoreline to sandy dunes. He'd stop midstream to give me bounty he had collected: shells, coins, pieces of glass, then continue his back-and-forth quest. I remember looking at all these tiny trinkets and laughing. Sam didn't need me to toss out shiny dimes. He had figured out all on his own that sparkling little treasures make walking even more fun.

I love reading, playing games, making crafts with our grandsons, but most of all I love walking with them. And just being together.

After dinner we watched the NY Yankee baseball game in our family room. Flip put his head on my lap and asked me to massage his back. We relaxed. My hand gently rubbing his back. My heart filling with joy. I probably would not have many more opportunities like this. I savor every fleeting grandson moment.

We planned, packed, and panicked as we navigated the daunting visa process. And then it was time to fly! We drove to Orlando, flew to Chicago, boarded the plane for our 13-hour flight to Beijing, and settled in. Jonathan by the window, me on the aisle, Flip in the middle.

After dinner, Flip explored his goodie bag. I bought a few books for him. He started with *Where is the Great Wall?* Jonathan had packed snacks. I brought the NY Yankee travel pillows I had made for each of them. I also created a list of common Mandarin words so we could at least learn to say "Hello—*Ni Hao*" and "Thank you—*Xie xie*." We practiced our words for a few minutes.

Jonathan propped his pillow by the window and promptly fell asleep. Flip leaned against Jonathan's shoulder for a while, then put his head on my lap, then back on Jonathan's shoulder. I knew I would not sleep much. For the first 6-7 hours I was content reading, relaxing, reflecting.

I watched Jonathan and Flip sleeping soundly and thought about how different my role would be on this trip compared to my trips to Peru with Rachel. In Peru, she and I expanded our mother-daughter relationship with its myriad of nuances. We added new roles of adult daughter traveling with her active, aging mom, exploring new terrain.

On our China trip, I would be Jonathan's mom and Flip's grandma. Different territory. New roles. *I'm excited about hiking on the Great Wall and exploring Beijing. But most of my joy will come from sharing this time with my son and grandson, enjoying these new wonders with them.*

I reviewed the itinerary. All we had tomorrow was a three-mile preview walk to help us understand what it would be like to run or walk on the Great Wall a few days later.

I closed my eyes and relaxed with a calming mantra: *Arrive in China, sleep a little, ride a bus, sit and listen, ride another bus, walk three miles, eat lunch, ride another bus back to the hotel. It will be fine.* When I opened my eyes, I realized I had slept for almost three hours!

By the time we landed, navigated customs, shuttled, arrived at the hotel, and plopped in bed, it was 11:00 p.m.

We got up at 2:30 the next morning and boarded the bus at 4:30. The big bus with 40 passengers weaved its way through busy Beijing streets, sped along a superhighway, then ambled along country roads. Three hours flew by. Jonathan napped. Flip took pictures out the window. "I'm glad you're taking so many pictures," I said. "I'm not sure what I expected, but I'm surprised to see so many mountains, lakes, and interesting trees."

"Thanks, Grandma. Most kids in my class will never get to come here, so I want to take pictures and show them as much as I can. And I can use them for my report." *Such a practical and thoughtful 10-year-old.*

We drove through Huangyaguan village and into a huge parking lot already filling with other buses. Then walked into the courtyard and were greeted by a giant yin-yang symbol painted on the block floor.

That yin-yang symbol would end up representing many light and dark facets of our trip. I needed to recognize that delicate balance. While we would see a bright and beautiful vision of China, this gilded picture would not represent reality for many who live here.

Each destination, no matter where I travel, has its dark side. Even the beautiful Grand Canyon usurped and ignored the rights of its original inhabitants, the Havasupai. I won't dwell on the darkness in China, but I *will* acknowledge its reality.

I looked up to the top of the tall block courtyard wall on the left and there it was: the Great Wall. Not what I expected! Not a tall flat monolithic barrier, but more like a snake slithering up and down the contours of the terrain, its bright earth tones glowing in the rising sun. It zigged and zagged up to little watch towers, then ducked down into valleys before stretching back up to another watch tower.

"Oh look, Grandma! It's the Great Wall!" said Flip. He jumped up on the bench to take pictures as the courtyard bleachers filled with more than a thousand people streaming in from the other buses. Some came in teams from multiple countries, speaking different languages. Athletes arrived in all different shapes and sizes. Five women walked in together wearing purple T-shirts with *Tanzania* emblazoned in white across their chests. Some athletes looked like they could be marching in the Olympic opening ceremony. There were also many ordinary-looking folks like us.

We sat, watched, and waited. Our 9:00 a.m. start time came and went. Finally, a young man, maybe the race director, walked up to the microphone. "Some buses were delayed. We will have to wait 60 to 90 minutes until they get here so we can give final instructions and updates. We have some water and snacks available over by the east wall. Please help yourselves. Please be patient."

The buses finally arrived. The same young man approached the microphone. "Thank you for your patience. We have several important announcements. Please listen carefully. The temperatures are typically in the mid-to-low eighties, but they have spiked into the nineties and may be even higher on event day. It's also unusually humid."

He paused, then continued, "Our event coordinators have decided that for the *first time ever*, we will allow participants to drop their registration to a lower level, either half marathon or 8.5K, with no penalties. Your safety is of utmost importance. This course is extremely challenging under the best of conditions. Please consider this option while you go on your preview walk and let us know if you want to drop to a lower level when you return.

"For today's walk you will ride a bus up the mountain to the Great Wall entrance. On Saturday the event will start right here at Yin-Yang Square. No bus ride. Just your own two feet. When everyone returns here today, we will serve a late lunch and get you on your buses back to your hotel so you can arrive in time for dinner around 6:00."

We finally boarded the waiting buses, rode up the mountain, and arrived at the Great Wall entrance at 12:30, more than three hours later than the planned start, and with more than a thousand other participants crowding onto the wall.

Time for another self-pep talk. *This is just three miles today. It's hot and humid. You're jetlagged and a little low on nutrition and hydration. Not a big deal. The big deal is that you are with your son and grandson on the Great Wall of China!*

Jonathan, Flip, and I stepped aside to let others rush by. Most ran. We took our time walking, climbing, taking pictures, soaking it all in, turning every which way. We saw offshoots of the wall in one direction, a steep stairway leading up to a regal watch tower crowned with parapets behind us. This section of the wall was restored with sturdy walls on each side, even handrails in some places.

After about 15 minutes, we saw people slowing down on a long flight of steps leading up to another watch tower ahead. As we walked forward, the bottleneck of participants stretched back to meet us like a slow-moving caterpillar. They stopped. We stopped. Five minutes, ten minutes, fifteen. Our supply of water was getting low. I chewed a few salt sticks and said, "I'm fine. Just a little dizzy. This is a perfect opportunity to sit on a step on the Great Wall and enjoy the view."

"Good idea! I'll sit with you," said Flip. We sat, enjoying the sights. "This is a moment, isn't it, Grandma?" Flip grinned.

Jonathan snaked ahead through the crowd to the aid station and came back with two water bottles and an update. "They're running out of water. The watch tower is mobbed. It has little alcoves with tiny open windows on each side and people are lining up to take selfies. We might as well sit here and let the crowd thin out."

A few minutes later, Jonathan said, "Mom, I'm going to switch from the marathon to the Fun Run. I'm not sure I could handle this heat. But more importantly, I don't want to leave you two alone to deal with something like this on Saturday. It will be less congested, but it will still be hot, probably hotter than today."

"Hon," I said, "I hoped you'd at least cut back to the half marathon because of the heat, but I hate it that you're doing the 8.5K because you're worried about me."

"I didn't brag to too many people about doing the marathon, not sure I could make it anyway. And now I can use my weak elderly mom as an excuse!" Jonathan grinned, then put his hand over his heart and looked up at the sky. "I'm not a wimp. I'm simply a kind and noble person doing what any good son would do." Flip giggled as he watched his dad hamming it up.

Jonathan locked eyes with me. "Mom, it will be cool for the three of us to walk together on Saturday. The thrill of the marathon got us here, but now we can turn this into a fun family adventure. All the pressure is off. Okay?"

"Okay," I smiled. The bottleneck eventually cleared. We finished our walk, savoring every step.

The next day was more relaxing with a later start. Our breakfast at the hotel included omelets and unique treats like steamed buns. Flip loved the deep-fried bread twists. We drank coffee and orange juice, then headed out to our bus for a full day of sightseeing led by our capable tour guide, Jenny: petite, 30ish, cute. She wore her long brown hair in a ponytail and laughed a lot, happily combining her knowledge of China with her own personal stories, using our travel time on the bus to share background, insights, and instructions.

We made a quick stop at a pearl *factory,* which consisted of a demonstration of opening a clam and finding a pearl followed by ample time in a giant pearl warehouse. Then we rode to the Summer Palace on dull gray highways lined with flower gardens—brilliant splashes of color, often in geometric designs—all works of beautiful botanical art.

"You will have one hour to walk around and see the sights in this section that includes the Hall of Benevolence and Longevity," Jenny instructed. "We will meet back here. I'll answer any questions and we will walk together to the next section. Please check your watches and return to this spot promptly in one hour."

The pavilion was surrounded by several bright red, intricately decorated buildings with open doors we could peer into. Giant sculptures filled the center courtyard. Lush greenery surrounded the building complex. It was beautiful, but I didn't feel my usual heartfelt tug until I saw Jonathan and Flip zipping around, peeking into the openings, shouting to each other and to me: "Look at this. Look at that! Mom, let's get a selfie in front of this gigantic vase."

"Okay! Then let me take a picture of you and Flip in front of this bronze beast with the dragon head," I said, overjoyed to see they were embracing this experience.

We joined Jenny and the group and walked along the lake front to the next section. "Please take your time to walk through the Long Corridor that is decorated with 14,000 intricate paintings. We will meet for lunch in 90 minutes over by the Marble Boat," said Jenny as she pointed to her map.

"You two go ahead. I want to spend a little more time looking at a few of these paintings," I said.

As Jonathan and Flip turned to go, they saw a group of seniors dressed in red performing Tai Chi in an open garden arena. "Hey, Grandma, are you going to join them?" Flip laughed. My family loves to tease me when they see me doing my little Tai Chi routine each morning as I wait for my English muffins in the toaster.

Jonathan smiled, "You're not going to cry, are you? I know how much you wanted to see some Tai Chi during our trip."

He knew this was a big moment for me, so they walked ahead, and I stood still appreciating the familiar grace and beauty, feeling the peace and joy of my classes back home. *I recognize some of these poses!* I thought to myself. *I know what this feels like, this standing meditation.* I watched a while longer, breathing deeply, feeling that incredible infusion of serenity as I moved my fingers to mimic their poses. *Relax, relax, relax.*

I strolled through the Long Corridor marveling at the array of fascinating paintings, then went to find the guys. "Hi, Mom," Jonathan said. "I got us some more water and we decided to sit on this wall and wait for Jenny. Have you noticed how people keep pointing at us?"

I responded, "I think they're looking at Flip."

Just then a young woman walked up and gestured that she wanted to have her picture taken with Flip. I shook my head no and was immediately sorry. She looked devasted. We walked over to meet Jenny. "Why are people pointing at Flip?" Jonathan asked her. "My mom just broke some girl's heart because she wouldn't let her take her picture with Flip," he laughed.

"Oh right. Your son is an oddity here," Jenny explained. "Many of the tourists you see here are from other parts of China and they have never seen a Caucasian child before. Having their picture taken with him would be like having a picture taken with a celebrity. Don't feel bad. There will be lots of opportunities to let other people take Flip's picture."

During our bus ride over to Old Beijing, the next stop on the tour, we drove by more beautiful strips of floral gardens. The color and artistry of each area was captivating, reinforcing the power of journeys, the paths we take getting to our next destination.

Jenny instructed, "You can take a short leisurely walk through these ancient neighborhoods. However, it's also an excellent opportunity to support our hard-working bikers who will pull your rickshaw. They are well-trained, safety certified, and take you through busy streets filled with shops and tea houses. You will have the opportunity to look down many *hutongs,* narrow alleys lined on either side with our traditional tiny courtyard homes. These neighborhoods existed in most of Beijing many years ago. Now there are just a few left, preserved as part of our history.

"The homes and courtyards are grey. From the outside they look the same; however, each courtyard and home interior is filled with brilliant colors and uniquely personal decorations of each inhabitant," Jenny added.

The rickshaws were lined up on the street. Flip and I climbed into one, and Jonathan into another right behind us. When the road curved, he exclaimed, "Grandma, look at all the rickshaws in front and behind us. It's like we're in a rickshaw parade!" He waved at some of the people on the sidewalks. They waved back, matching his grin. Flip's delight was contagious.

I relaxed and enjoyed the sights and sounds. One side of the street was filled with animated crowds, tea houses, and shops. On the other side were those narrow alleys Jenny had described. I tried imagining the unique beauty of each compact courtyard and home. For a moment, my mind traveled back to all the tiny places we had lived growing up. It didn't matter how small: a teardrop trailer parked in someone's back yard, the apartment where Mom slept on the couch and hung a sheet down the middle of the one bedroom so Chuck and I could each have our private space. She always planted morning glories along the omnipresent chicken wire fences. Those flowers welcomed us with their cascade of colors every morning. We learned to live small *and* beautifully.

We rode by a lake, serenaded by the music of bird songs and the clattering of the black narrow rickshaw wheels on the concrete road. When we arrived at the end, Flip took the money Jonathan had given him and handed it to the driver saying, "*Xie, xie.*" It was hot. This man had worked so hard. He nodded and gave Flip a tired smile. Then he rushed over and pulled his rickshaw back in line waiting for the next riders.

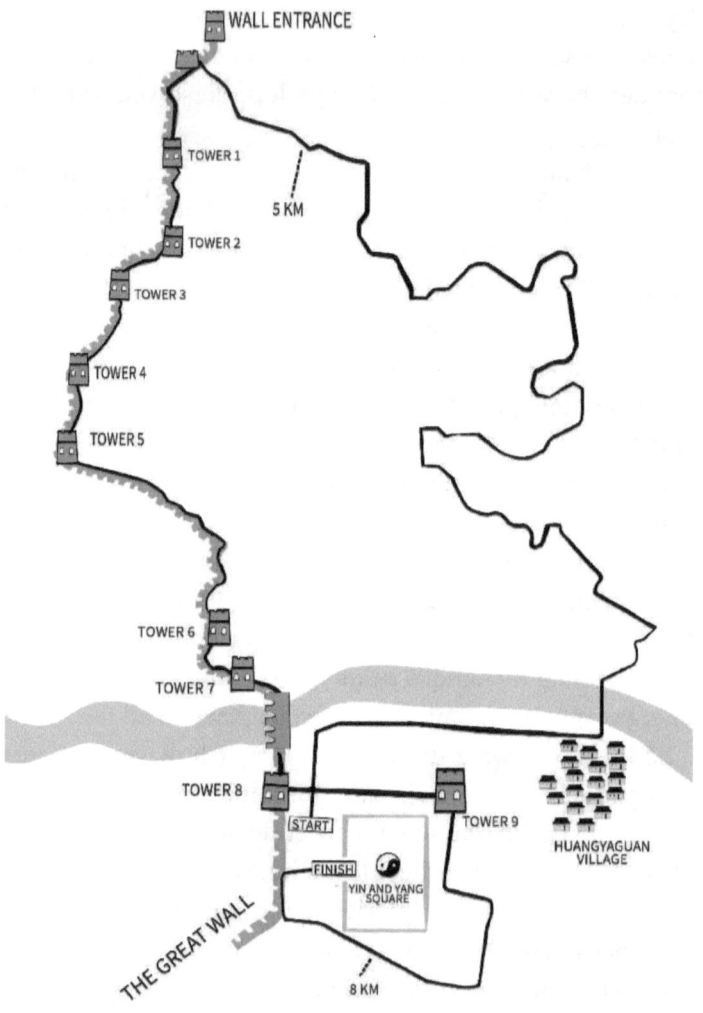

Later we went to the hotel ballroom for a carb-load pre-race buffet dinner. The master of ceremonies called for attention and gave instructions. "All three groups (marathon, half marathon, and

8.5K) will start their race at the square, run through town and up the mountain for the first three miles. No bus rides up the hill tomorrow! It will be another very hot day. Please stay hydrated. Shortly after the fourth water stop you will arrive at the Great Wall and will continue your run for 3.5K (2.2 miles) before returning to the square where the Fun Run will end."

Jonathan and I clicked our glasses of water together in a quick toast, looked at each other, and smiled with relief as the speaker continued to give detailed instructions and warnings to the full and half marathoners.

The air was already heating up when we climbed on our bus early the next morning. After our three-hour drive, we returned to the beautiful courtyard with the Great Wall looming up and down the mountains. Our Fun Run plans left us feeling festive and relaxed as we walked around the square, taking pictures, then posing by the yin-yang symbol. The first two waves headed out. We lined up at the back of Fun Runners.

We headed out of the courtyard, then turned right and started to walk through the main street of Huangyaguan Village. The staging area had been quiet, so we were surprised when we walked out of the square into a blast of cheers. People were lined along both sides of the road. Many of them started pointing at Flip, taking pictures, calling at him to look at them. Jenny had told us Flip was a bit of a celebrity, but I was shocked. And Flip was scared.

He started to cry and ran back to his dad who was walking behind us taking pictures. We stepped to the side of the road. Flip sobbed. Jonathan bent down, clutched Flip's shoulders as he talked intently, quietly. He pointed to the crowd along the road. Flip looked, nodded, calmed down, wiped his eyes and nose, and headed back to me.

"You okay, hon?"

He murmured, "Yes. I was just upset that people were taking pictures of me, and they weren't even asking permission. I mean, it's not like I'm some reality star or something." (I smothered my smile.) "Dad talked to me. I'm okay now."

He walked ahead and even stepped over to the crowd and lifted his hand so they could high-five him. Others ran up with their hands lifted. Phone cameras snapped. Flip turned, gave me a little smile, and we continued walking up the road as the crowds thinned out. We turned left and walked up the incline.

The road up the mountain was more pleasant than we expected. On Thursday's bus ride, it didn't register that most of this portion was shaded. We walked by a little village on the right side with views of the Great Wall meandering along the mountain top on the left side. "Why don't you and Flip sit on those rocks so I can get a picture of you with the wall in the background? We have the time. We are in no rush," said Jonathan.

As we posed for our picture, I said, "You know, Flip, I never expected to see the Great Wall go up and down hills with so many steps and guard houses."

Flip agreed, "And I really did not expect to see the wall dip so low and close to the ground. When we walked on Thursday, I loved seeing those people on horses, just riding along the wall almost right beside us. I could have reached out and petted one of those horses! Did you get a picture?"

"No, but I'll be sure to take one of you standing on that spot today. Your dad will probably take even more pictures today too. He's sure having fun. I'm glad we're doing this together."

Shortly after passing the 5k mark, we climbed up the steps to the entrance of the Huangyaguan section of the Great Wall. We walked and chatted with some of the other slow walkers. It was hot with no shade. As Flip and I climbed up one long flight of uneven stairs, he offered, "Grandma, you can put your hand on my shoulder if that makes you feel more comfortable. Some of these steps are steep."

"Thanks, hon, I will!" I responded, appreciating his steady assistance and the sweet touch of his strong boney little shoulder.

Another moment. Another precious connection.

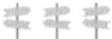

Jonathan caught up with us just as we reached another landing and Flip asked, "Dad, is it okay if I run ahead up to that next guard house? I promise to stay there and not go any farther."

"Sure! Have fun. Be careful and wave when you get there," said Jonathan.

Flip tore off, running up the steps.

Jonathan burst out laughing, "Look at that kid, he's really got the spirit now."

"What did you say to him that helped turn him around?" I asked. "He was pretty upset with all that attention when we started the race."

"I just told him to look at people's faces, how happy they were to see someone like him," Jonathan answered. "He promised me he would try to be friendly even though it still made him feel uncomfortable. And now look at him!" Jonathan chuckled.

Jonathan shook his head. "This heat must be beating those marathoners up. I bet many of them don't make the cut-off time. I could not have done it. But, of course, the main reason will always be that I was taking care of good old mom," he laughed. He offered his arm when the uneven steps got steeper and added, "This is much more fun. We're practically alone strolling, stopping whenever we want, taking our time on the Great Wall of China. We made it our very own Fun Walk."

Just then, Flip popped out of the guard house high on the hill ahead and gestured for us to hurry up. A blue-suited guard was standing with him, her hand on his shoulder. Jonathan said, "Hey Mom, do you mind if I run up and see what's going on?"

"Of course not! Go ahead." Jonathan ran up the steps and disappeared into the watch tower. I kept climbing, then heard Jonathan's raucous laugh, that kind that makes you join in even if you don't know what's so funny.

"Everything is fine, Mom. You have to see this," Jonathan called. By the time I got close I could see tears running down his cheeks. He explained as I stepped into the dark interior, "They are shutting down this water station and wanted to get a picture with Flip before they left."

We walked through the stone watch tower toward the small arched opening on the opposite end where Flip was standing, smiling, clutching a bottle of water. He was flanked by two tall, slender, young, official-looking aid-station workers, dressed in blue, trying to look serious. The woman we saw earlier stood behind Flip, her hands resting on his shoulders, leaning to the side so her whole face could be in the picture. They were posing patiently, waiting for Jonathan to take pictures with each of their phones and then finally his own. Jonathan started taking pictures. The woman smiled big and even the two men popped a little grin.

"*Xie xie, Xie xie!*" They checked out their phones, packed up their stuff, and gave us each two bottles of water. They high-fived Flip and headed out, chattering and laughing.

"This was so cool," Flip exclaimed. "When I came in, they looked surprised and a little worried I was alone. So, I said, 'Daddy and Grandma' and took the woman out the back so I could point to you two. She nodded and gave me a thumbs up. They gave me some water and showed me different window openings where I could take pictures. Then they gestured, pointing to their phones that they wanted their picture taken with me since I'm such a celebrity," he said as he modestly cocked his head. "That's when I came out and called for you."

Jonathan grinned, "Now I know for sure my little talk did some good."

"You're right," Flip agreed. "I was pretty upset when we first started out, but I did just what you said and looked at their faces. What can I say, it made people happy to see me," Flip paused for a dramatic sigh, mimicking his dad. "So, I calmed down and it started to be fun. These guards were really nice. It was so cool we could understand each other mainly by gesturing."

Sweet little connection on the Great Wall. We will cherish both memories big and small.

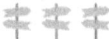

We passed through more watch towers, then descended a steep hill and arrived at the walls of the Huangyaguan Fortress. We crossed the 8.5K mark just before climbing down steps from the wall, returning to our familiar Yin and Yang Square, and crossing the finish line tired and triumphant.

As we waited for the marathoners to finish, Jonathan and Flip wandered around the courtyard, picking up snacks, laughing, and chatting with others. I sat in the bleachers watching them, determined to digest all the sights and sounds of this incredible ending. I didn't want to take pictures. I just wanted to capture all I could in my mind. *I need to embrace this moment so I can remember it forever.* My chest tightened. I took a deep breath and held back the tears.

Our event was relatively short, just a little more than five miles. But we had traveled such a great distance.

Flip learned the reciprocal joy of making others happy. Jonathan handled his *generational sandwich role* with impeccable grace and humor. He honed his teaching skills and taught Flip to look up and lean in. He supported me and shared the joy of cutting back and creating bigger rewards.

We would see and do many more things on this trip, but the finish line of our Fun Run was the grande finale. It was an ending to be savored and celebrated. It was the peak, summit, apex of our trip.

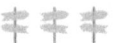

Our final two days in China provided our epilogue, yin and yang, dark and light—even wet. At Tiananmen Square, Jenny herded us together so we would join other groups led by a new guide. He quickly greeted us and quietly conveyed cryptic instructions. "It will be crowded, so please stick together. Security is extremely stringent here. It is not a place for joking around. You will see many uniforms, but there are also plain clothes military patrolling this area."

He continued, "Many of you want to know where the 'Tank Man Protester' stood in 1989. I can show you the spot, but I must speak in code. We will walk together. I will stop and say, 'This is a good place to see every section of the square.' When I say that, I will be standing in the exact spot where the protester stood. Please do not ask any questions. I could get in trouble. Just stand there quietly. Look around and move on."

We came to the spot. Stopped in silence. The sun blazed bright as we stood together, united in our compassion, honoring a man who had stood so strong, holding up his hand to halt injustice.

As instructed, we moved on in a sad haze. Then we rejoined Jenny and were herded together for a team photo in front of the iconic red wall with the gigantic picture of Mao Zedong.

We stood at the entrance of the Forbidden City. "As soon as you enter this complex you will see five white bridges. Now listen carefully," Jenny had relaxed. Her humor had returned. We all relaxed a bit too.

She lifted her head, adding a bit of drama to her next announcement. "This is your unique opportunity to be infused with the five virtues of benevolence, righteousness, generosity, intelligence, and fidelity preached by Confucius." She let this sink in. "All you have to do is walk over each of the five white bridges you will encounter on the other side of this red wall." Another long pause. "But you can walk *only* one way on each one. If you walk back and forth, you will wipe out your new virtue," Jenny said with a grin.

Armed with our new knowledge, Jonathan, Flip, and I walked through the massive archway leading to this ancient world. We followed Jenny's instructions and walked over each of the five bridges. Only one way over each. Then on the final bridge, we paused, taking a selfie and basking in our virtuosity. As I stood there between Jonathan and Flip, I imagined my own sixth bridge with the virtue of balance. I was playing three roles: Self, Mom, and Grandma, savoring my contented equilibrium.

On our last tour day, we paused in the center of a courtyard surrounded by the glorious celestial structures of the Temple of Heaven: tall circular buildings covered in intricate paintings with parapets that soared up to the firmament.

Suddenly the sky opened and unleashed an unexpected shower creating another memorable family moment. We did not run for cover or even dive into a gift shop for umbrellas. We had so little time with much more to see. So, we stayed in the courtyard. Jonathan stood facing up to the sky with his arms out, fingers pinched and palms facing upward, catching the rain.

Flip giggled. "Oh, Grandma. Look at Dad," he said shaking his head. The world paused. Jonathan held his pose. Flip's mouth stayed open in a big laugh. In slow-motion, rain drops slowly splashed on leaves, sprang up and down, and smashed on the ground. Just a moment. One more. I blinked, and the normal speed of life returned as we stood in the rain, enjoying the soft patter of flowers bobbing.

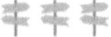

On our final and blissfully calm morning, Jonathan said, "Mom, I really want you to see where Flip and I went on our early morning walks while you were getting ready. We still have time before the airport shuttle."

Jonathan led us off the beaten path and into a place that seemed hidden from tourists just a few steps from our hotel. We crossed a pedestrian bridge over a busy highway and entered a world of narrow streets like those on our Old Beijing rickshaw tour. Food shops perched along main streets and stretched down the alleys. People stood outside cooking on open grills. A few customers sat at outside tables eating, but food was also piling up on big tables, almost like an assembly line.

"Look, those are the bread twists like we ate for breakfast at the hotel," exclaimed Flip. "We get to see where they are made. How cool!" A sweet way to end our trip.

Our trip to China created a new experience to cherish forever and added another lovely dimension of travel. There will be other roles in future trips along with opportunities to enhance my perspective, increase adaptability, and strengthen relationships.

Playing different roles in my trips does not mean I have to *juggle* them. That suggests a level of stress and fear that something might get dropped. Playing different roles for me will achieve balance—*alignment*—calm and smooth like a meditative Tai Chi routine.

.

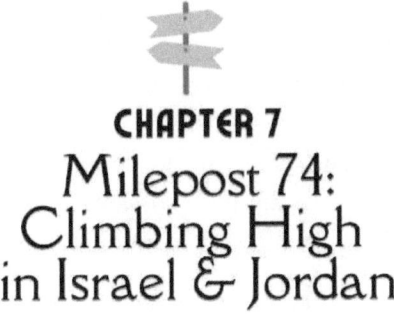

CHAPTER 7

Milepost 74:
Climbing High
in Israel & Jordan

"I can't get to the airport! That Pacific Ocean hurricane flooded the entire west side of Phoenix. My Lyft driver just called. He can't get to my address," Sherry gasped. "I don't know what to do. I'm checking the roads, but it doesn't look good. I don't think I'll be able to get out on this flight and meet you at JFK. I can't afford to change flights, so I may not be able to go to Israel with you. Please go, Sandi. I'll keep you posted."

"Okay, Sherry. I'm so sorry! Remember we have flight insurance to cover things like this. We can figure things out even if we can't fly together," I quickly reply before she clicks off. Then I text her, "Please text me and call Arnie if I don't respond."

"What happened?" Arnie heard my side of the call. "Is that Sherry? What's going on?"

I had been up since 4:30, extra early so I wouldn't have to rush to get ready for my driver to Jacksonville airport. Just before Sherry's call, I was sitting in Arnie's office, enjoying our peaceful, parting time together, doing my best to avoid my usual manic pre-trip hysteria. Passport? Check. Flight times? Check. Confirmation from my driver? Check. It was October 2018, and up until this point, most of our Israel travel plans had worked out well. But now this?

"She's flooded in and may not get to the airport in time. If she misses her flight, she can probably fly out later today or tomorrow. But she says she may not be able to make it at all."

"Go," Arnie quickly responded. "Just do it. You have everything planned. You want to do this. You will be with others on the tour even if Sherry can't make it. It will be an adventure. I know how much you like to take time to process new information and avoid last-minute decisions. But you should not miss this." I knew I could depend on Arnie to encourage and give me the support I needed to live my travel dreams.

I wanted more time to decide, but I wanted to go on this trip even more.

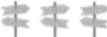

Sherry had encouraged me to ask for a wheelchair at JFK since I had such a short time to make my connection. I hated to play the age card at just 74, but I was pretty sure I could not make it on my own.

Good decision! I reached the boarding area with just minutes to spare. The young man who pushed my wheelchair said, "You are almost 75, traveling alone for the first time on an international flight. You earned this. It's my pleasure to help you get started on your big trip."

Sherry's text pops up. "Getting things resolved with the insurance company. I will meet you in Tel Aviv."

I settle into my aisle seat and take a deep breath. *This is good.* Maybe everything will work out after all.

Then it isn't good. After my 8-hour flight, I enter the Rome terminal at 2:30 am. I had expected things to be quiet at this time of day, but not silent. All the other passengers head out the exits. The signs are all dark. No flight information. I am alone. The other passageways are blocked. *Calm down*, I say to myself. *Absolutely no reason to expect every airport will be the same as those in the states.* I decide to sit and wait.

I start to get nervous but talk myself down again. *I have a two-hour layover. I won't panic for at least another hour.* I sit, try to read, give up, look up. A few travelers walk in and quickly leave through the exits. Then a few more enter, stand, and look around. I gather up my stuff and walk over. "Are you flying to Tel Aviv?" I'm not sure they understand me. They shake their heads. Then they sit down. Okay. *When in Rome.* I sit back down too.

Then 30-40 people flood the airport, splashing through the aisles in roaring waves. They don't leave. They stay. They stand. Some sit. They talk loudly, full of excitement and passion. I see beards, tall dark hats, black coats, head scarves, long dresses. It wasn't the Cavalry. It was even better. It was Chabad—the sect of Judaism dedicated to teaching and outreach with a strong presence in Israel. *Yes, of course. Oh, happy day.* I walk up to one of the women and ask, "Are you going to Israel?"

She smiles. "Yes, of course." To her credit, she didn't ask, *What was your first clue?* She continues, "We are coming home from a Chabad convention in New York. Are you flying to Tel Aviv?"

"Yes. It's my first trip. I didn't see any flight information, so I wasn't sure I was in the right place."

"You are. Just follow us and you'll be fine. Are you Jewish?"

"Yes," I nod. "Thank you so much for your help."

"I have something for you," she says as she rummages in her purse. She takes out a little packet, presses it into my hands, looks long into my eyes, and with a little smile says, "Enjoy your stay in Israel."

She turns to join the other ladies in the group. I sit back down and open the packet. It is a small teaching kit with two small Shabbat candles, traditionally lit at sunset on Friday to welcome the Jewish Sabbath. I smile. "Yes, of course."

The terminal lights up. Flight information flashes on the screens. It starts to look like a *normal* terminal. Everyone heads toward a boarding gate that is suddenly staffed. Lines start moving. I dig out my passport and boarding pass, grab my purse and backpack, and join the crowd.

When we land, I check into the Dan Panorama Hotel around noon Tel Aviv time, 6:00 a.m. Florida time. More than twenty-four hours, no sleep, sore, exhausted, even discouraged. I take a vow: *Never again. I'm too old for this.*

By the time I wake up from my short nap, I'm ready to do some exploring. My psyche is also refreshed. Instead of even considering, *Never again,* I'm reframing my story. *I traveled more than twenty-four hours with no sleep, pain in both hips, all alone at 74. I got this!*

I walk across the street to the beach savoring the cool sea breeze and shimmering sun. I stop and stare. *There it is! That big blue oval I remember seeing in textbooks when I was in elementary school. How magnificent. What a moment!* I'm walking slowly but my pulse is racing. I am totally excited, but I resist the urge to yell out to people walking by, "Can you believe it? That is the Mediterranean Sea!"

I find a bench to sit and think about all that has happened so far. Decisions that worked out well, problems solved on my own, levels of confidence heightened, new muscles strengthened—especially from traveling alone without the comfort of a thought-partner. I am already enriched by my journey.

I watch runners, bikers, individuals, and families glide by looking serene and safe. It dawns on me I've seen no military presence yet. I touch the little yin-yang pendant on my necklace and think about past bombings and present beauty. When we started planning this trip I was scared. Then I acknowledged the danger and accepted reality. *There will always be a risk/reward balance no matter where we go. I will enjoy my time here, being cautious but not constrained.*

I think about another new role I will play on this trip. Sherry McClain is Arnie's cousin. We share some family events and history, but traveling together will be an entirely new experience. I'm not worried, just curious. I wonder how it will all work out.

We both wanted to pay extra to add a trip to Petra. We're both Jewish. She by birth. I by choice. We're both old. She's 18 months older and has more travel experience. I have more energy. We have adult children. Sherry's husband died a few years ago. We have confessed that at times we snore and give each other permission to reach over and nudge. That's about all I know so far. I'm sure we will learn much more during our ten days together.

I decide to wait until Sherry arrives to celebrate the beginning of our adventure together by dipping our toes in the Mediterranean Sea.

My single celebration has already begun. I have the luxury of time to explore on my own today. No schedule to dictate. Traveling alone is not nearly as intimidating as I thought it would be. *So, Sandi, what do you want to do?* It's supposed to be hot during most of our trip, so I will make the most of the shining sun and soft sea breezes that embrace me today.

Later I return to the hotel to check out the post cards at the gift shop. The shopkeeper takes charge. "Don't use the ATM here in the hotel and don't drop off your postcards at the front desk. I'll give you better locations for both. You can even buy your stamps from me, but it may take a few minutes to add them up since they're all lower denominations." I agree, stand at the counter, then wander around the gift shop, come back to the counter.

"Why don't you just give me enough stamps for ten postcards, and I'll come back later for the rest."

He keeps counting and stacking sometimes four different stamps to add up to the cost for one postcard, then waves his hand.

"Wait, wait just a few more minutes and I can get them all for you. What's your big hurry? Please be *pa-tient.*" He looks up, lifts his eyebrows, cocks his head, and grins.

I take a big breath, try hard to be *pa-tient,* then take another deep breath as he carefully counts out more than sixty stamps for my twenty postcards. Done. Finally! I smile and say, "Thank you, sir," returning his grin.

He nods his head, "Remember where the ATM and mailbox are located, and be sure to come back if you need more stamps. I have many more."

I check at the front desk. "Go to the Carmel Market. You may see a few markets like this during your tour, especially in Old Jerusalem, but our market is the best," advises the desk clerk with authority. How could I resist? I start walking. Fortuitously, the mailbox is on my way, and I get to walk through a lovely park filled with sturdy benches, stately statues, and canopied shade from sycamore and eucalyptus trees.

The Carmel Market is jammed with vibrant colorful stalls on either side of a narrow alley filled with everything in abundance. The baklava table has at least twenty different varieties. The bread table is piled high with braided challah and loaves of bread in multiple shapes and sizes. I pass by a date table, an olive table, and then come to a fresh-squeezed juice stand with what will become my go-to drink for the rest of the trip, carrot juice! I figure out how to use the ATM to retrieve shekels with a good exchange rate of more than three shekels to a dollar. I meander up and down the main section then weave through a few side paths where I discover a table filled with inexpensive intricately braided bracelets, perfect for little Hanukkah gifts.

The lunch counters are packed so I decide to head back to the hotel for a late snack before Sherry arrives. I'm not sure of her eating preferences, but just in case she might be tired and famished, I buy an extra serving of Israeli salad, hummus, and pita wedges and take it up to the room. She texts me when she lands so I head down to the lobby to meet her. We hug and hustle up to our room so she can shower, snack, and settle in.

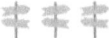

By the next morning, Sherry is willing to go for a short walk. Then she's ready to return to the hotel. "Go on, Sandi. I know you have a list of things you want to see. Enjoy! We'll catch up later."

"You sure?"

"I'm sure." Sherry turns back. I move forward.

A scattering of street vendors and food stalls in an open-air flea market fill the road with brilliant colors and the air with savory smells. On my left I see stone arches with narrow alleys quickly turning into stairs leading up the hill. *This is just the second day of my trip and I've already seen, done, and tasted so much, almost all on my own*, I marvel to myself. *And now I'm walking through the Old Jaffa Port built 4,000 years ago, the oldest port in the world.*

I watch a sailor standing in his small boat mending his nets and imagine Jonah getting ready to head out on his tiny craft to meet his destiny with the whale. I pause to let that history flood my head and heart and then start looking for the two other things on my list: the old lighthouse and Clock Tower Square.

I turn back north, walking close to the shore side as I crane my neck looking up above the tall buildings that line the street. I finally see the lighthouse perched on a hilltop hovering high on a hill behind a mosque. Red and white stripes, only 30 feet tall. The lamp tips sideways. Its guard rails are broken, falling in pieces. It was built in 1865, just a few years older than the St Augustine Lighthouse that was built between 1871 and 1874. But, unlike St. Augustine, this one was deactivated in 1966 and quickly fell into disrepair. While I'm sad to see it struggle to survive, I'm glad to know it's still used as a daytime navigational aid by those at sea. I look up and whisper, "Thank you for your service, dear lighthouse."

I climb a few flights of steep stairs up to another street level, searching for the next thing on my list, and there it is: the Clock Tower! It's hard to believe so much history could be contained in a single elegant monolith. This tall limestone structure has two clocks, Ottoman architecture arches, and a unique steeple. I had read its stories and now I get to meet it in person.

I return to the hotel, reunite with Sherry, and we walk across the beach down to the shore. A young girl kindly takes our pictures as we dip our toes into the Mediterranean Sea, our official welcome to Israel.

"Now that we have our pictures, let's just stand, let the water splash our legs, and appreciate this moment," I tell Sherry. "I can get so caught up with checking things off my list and taking pictures that sometimes I forget to fully embrace the moment. I'm trying to be more intentional about pausing and appreciating this trip, especially since there will be so many things to see and do."

Sherry bursts out laughing. "I already figured that out! I'm not sure I can slow you down, but I'll try. I love your passion, energy, and enthusiasm, but I think I might have one thing that will help. Remember that story you told me about how you were getting antsy waiting for the clerk to figure out all your postcard stamps? He said, 'Please be *pa-tient*.'"

"Oh yes," I laugh. "Perfect! If you see me getting a little frantic, you can just say, 'Sandi, please be *pa-tient*.'"

"I'm already delighted to be traveling with you," I said, putting my hand on Sherry's shoulder. "You didn't give up. You worked through the delays and trip insurance hassle and managed to get here. And, today, when you got tired, you were honest with yourself and with me. You knew it was time to call it quits. There have been times when my walking or hiking buddy gets overwhelmed but then keeps pushing until she gets grumpy, injured, or ill. You didn't do any of that. I can trust you to be honest. Thank you! That means so much."

Sherry smiles. "I'm guessing both of us will have a pretty long gratitude list by the time this trip is over."

We walk back to our room for the night.

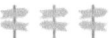

This will be my first multi-day bus trip with an itinerary packed with tour stops and items of interest. There will be big stops and little stops. *I will enjoy the little ones and totally embrace the big ones,* I pledge to myself. *I do not want to feel overwhelmed at the end of each day and at the end of this trip. I want to feel enlightened and entranced with a few experiences I will treasure forever.*

The next day we travel north along the coast, making many quick stops and ending the morning at the border of Israel and Lebanon, two countries that are long-time foes and still formally at war. Sherry and I stand just a few feet away from the heavily guarded check point as we get a quick geography lesson from a large sign with arrows pointing south to Jerusalem (205 miles) and north to Beirut (120 miles).

We walk back a stone's throw to enter a cable car that takes us down to the geological miracle of the Rosh Hanikra Grottos, large sea caves formed by thousands of years of the Mediterranean Sea smashing against the soft chalk rock at the base of towering cliffs.

I step into the grotto and listen to the crashing waves. I walk a few steps on the damp uneven path and see a small alcove off to the right with a large opening facing a brilliant turquoise pond. The blue waters resemble the other-worldly ponds at Havasupai Falls at the bottom of the western end of the Grand Canyon. I step forward to get a better look. It's not crowded, so I can stand for a few minutes letting the azure beauty seep in. I catch up with Sherry who is staying on the main path, then head off into another alcove for another spectacular view. "I never knew what a grotto was and now I have walked through one!"

Soon we turn south to another stop that will definitely be on my top ten list. In high school, I read *Exodus* by Leon Uris with its stories of kibbutzim, the early collective agricultural communities scattered across Israel. Our destination, Kibbutz Lavi, was founded in 1951 and originally included children who had been evacuated from Germany as part of the Kindertransport program created before the Holocaust. In addition to agriculture, it became a producer of carpentry products for synagogues and has even added a hotel that will serve as our home base for the next two nights.

We step off the bus and are greeted by our local host with an enticing invitation. "You will have almost 90 minutes after dinner and before our evening presentation. Please take advantage of this time to walk around and enjoy our campus. Most of our 150 families will be eating a dinner of leftovers from yesterday's buffet meal that was served here at the hotel. We are a cooperative, communal community. We share and contribute to the best of our ability, and we make best use of the food we grow in our fields and gardens."

After dinner, Sherry opts to sit in the lounge and jot notes in her journal. I happily accept the host's invitation to go out and explore the campus. After collegial chaos of touring with a busload of people all day, this stroll is a respite. At first, I'm excited that I can finally add reality to my imagined pictures of a living, working kibbutz. I'm all alone. It's dark. I consider turning back to the hotel. Then shake off the fear, knowing this short self-tour will educate and inspire me. I won't regret this.

I turn onto a softly lit tree-lined path. Many families are sitting out on the porches of their tiny homes eating their evening meal. Ambient sounds of quiet conversation drift into the calm and peaceful atmosphere. It's like listening to a choir of melodic children's voices syncopated with low-pitched adult chants.

I visit the small synagogue, a holy place filled with pews and other sanctuary furniture constructed by the residents of this community. I step back outside and walk in the cloistered beauty of narrow paths lined by flowers and shrubs, accented by tiny lights. I return to the main street, then enter a dark memorial garden sprinkled with lights that illuminate plaques telling stories. The serenity of this sanctuary seeps into my soul. I pause. I sit. Reflect. Then it's time to head back to the hotel for the evening presentation.

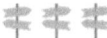

The next morning we're back on the bus for a day trip. Mali, our tour guide, is a *Sabra*, someone born in Israel, and former member of the Israeli army. She is young, passionate, full of knowledge, and understandably biased in her view of Israel. She smiles. She talks. She listens. She has already learned our names.

Although I hate to make special requests, I take the plunge. "Mali, I understand this is a tour and you have boundaries and restrictions, but is it at all possible for me to hike up the Snake Path at Masada, even if I skip the tour at the top?"

Mali looks crushed. "Oh, Sandi, I wish I could, but our insurance and the tight schedule don't allow that hike. I am so sorry."

"It's totally fine. I figured that might be the case, but I had to ask," I tell her. "That curving trail from the base of the mountain all the way up to the top looks so intimidating and inviting. I just want to take every opportunity to push myself to try new things, even if they are a bit scary."

Mali's eyes twinkle and she grins. "If you really like doing things that are a little frightening, be sure to swim in the natural pond when we visit Gan HaShlosha National Park. The pond is so deep and dark you can't see the bottom, and it's full of fish that will hit your feet as they slither through the cool water. Locals enjoy this opportunity to relax and rejuvenate, but most people on my tours won't consider this. If you can build up the nerve to take the plunge, you won't forget or regret it."

"Okay. Thanks," I say with a smile. *Yikes*. I think. *Hiking, climbing, and walking are easy and fun for me. Swimming is not. I struggle, flail, and feel like I'm losing my breath. But I promised myself I'd take advantage of every opportunity to try new things and step out of my comfort zone during each of my trips. I need to do this. Even if I don't want to.*

"So, you really like hiking and climbing?" Mali says.

"I do, but it's really fine," I reassure her. "You give us many opportunities to walk around and I'm sure there will even be a little climbing when we get to Masada."

The next day we stop at the Beit She'an National Park, a vast complex of colonnaded streets, temples, and theaters of an ancient Greek city. The site is filled with dozens of standing fragments of structures, almost all white, entirely beautiful. I see a high fortification hill just beyond the complex. My eyes immediately focus on a tiny set of black metal steps *snaking* all the way up to the top. I squint my eyes. The steps even have railings.

Mali watches me study that hill, then she gathers the group together around a large table. "Today, I will give you a choice. You may listen to my *very interesting* lecture as we stand around this model of the city." She pauses and looks at me. "Or you may go off on your own to climb those 150 steps up to the top of that lookout hill. You will not hurt my feelings if you opt for the climb. Just be sure you're back here in 45 minutes to get back on the bus."

Sherry smiles. She knows what's coming. "Go! I'll fill you in on anything you miss in the lecture. Have fun."

"Thank you, Sherry!" One couple and I raise our hands and we head for the hills. We three stick together as we climb up the rickety metal staircase all the way to the top. What a sight! We explore little buildings and monuments not visible from the bottom. The couple heads down so they can catch the final portion of Mali's lecture.

I linger at the top, inspecting and admiring the ancient fortifications. I stand to savor my bird's-eye view of the beautiful white ruins arrayed below.

Then, I rush down the steps, grasping the helpful railings, determined not to be late, and get to the bus just in time. "See, Sandi," Mali says. "I couldn't give you the Masada Snake Path, but I could give you Beit She'an!" I'm not sure which of us is happier. We grin big and high five.

The next day we stop at Gan HaShlosha National Park with the swimming *opportunity* Mali described.

My trepidation surges as I stand behind three men from our tour group. The first two slip comfortably into the water. (That's good.) The third dips his toe in and yells, "Fish are hitting my foot! No way!" He backs up and quickly retreats. (Not good.)

My turn. I step onto the steep ladder, take a deep breath, let go, and slip in, treading water so my head and hair stay high and dry. I flounder and blink at flashes of sunlight reflecting off silvery fish. I flip to a side stroke and lock my eyes on Sherry as she walks along the bank, waving, shouting encouragement, taking pictures.

It's not that far. Just a pool length. I manage to glide and kick forward, even enjoying the view. "You're almost there!" Sherry calls. I grab the ladder, climb up and out, catching my breath while Sherry cheers. Delighted I did it. Happy it's done. Knowing I will never regret taking the plunge.

Sherry helped me navigate through my fear across that pond. A few days later I could return the favor when she balks at floating in the Dead Sea. "You go ahead, Sandi. I'm just going into this indoor pool. It's the same water. It's just not as intimidating."

"And it also won't be nearly as momentous and memorable. I understand your fear, especially since Mali warned that we should not get any toxic water in our eyes or mouth." I pause, giving Sherry a minute. "Will you at least consider holding my hand and stepping into the shallow end of the Dead Sea with me?

The second it gets too overwhelming we'll stop and turn back. I promise you will not regret this." Sherry purses her lips, gives me a look, and reluctantly agrees.

We wade in. We float in the Dead Sea. She does not regret it.

After our water stop at Gan HaShlosha, we continue sitting together on the bus heading south, sharing sweet time together. Sherry turns to me, "I know you have several things on your list, and I love that about you. I have one big thing on my list too. And I want your help." *Wow! I love this.* "You and Arnie were so close to my parents, especially when you lived in Tucson and I lived in Phoenix. It's almost like you adopted each other. They weren't ever alone or lonely. That meant so much to me." She looks down at her purse. "I keep a small vial of their ashes with me, and I'd like you to help me find a spot to scatter them somewhere on this trip. I have no idea where that will be, but I trust we will know it when we see it—when we feel it."

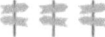

At sunset we stop at Mount Scopus for a ceremony to celebrate our arrival at Jerusalem, a place honored by Jews, Christians, and Muslims, and described as the holiest city in the world.

We enter the city limits and I immediately notice the heavy military presence. "They are so young!" I say to Sherry. "These are boys and girls. No. They are heavily armed soldiers. They don't look much older than our grandsons, Andrew and Jonathan."

There is heavy security, especially around Old City Jerusalem, but we feel secure, not scared. On our first night, Sherry and I wander down to Ben Yehuda Street to explore the shops, enjoy the lights and lively crowds, and eat a large serving of fudge gelato for dinner.

The next few days are filled with day trips from our Jerusalem home base. We tour Yad Vashem, the World Holocaust Remembrance Center. After spending hours in the Center, we still have ample time to sit on one of the benches by the tree garden to reflect, remember, and honor. The millions who perished. The righteous few who courageously acted to save others. A holy place.

During one of those day trips, we walk up the steep slope of Ammunition Hill, now a memorial site to those who perished in the battle for Jerusalem in the Six-Day War.

We climb a hill. I feel a soft earth shift and look ahead. "Sherry," I point. "That tree."

She stops, looks. "That's it, isn't it?" I nod, unable to speak. Sherry slowly opens her purse, reverently takes out the vial and sprinkles a few ashes. She hands the vial to me. I do the same. Then I hand it back to her so she can finish. *May their memory be a blessing.*

Shabbat rolls around and Sherry and I are ready for a day of walking, resting, with no bus rides and tours. Our hotel is just a half mile from Old City. We stroll through lovely, tree-lined neighborhoods to reach the Jaffa Gate of the Armenian Quarter. We navigate bustling alleys. We shop, sip our preferred juices of carrot and orange, and enjoy the smells and cacophony of the Christian and Armenian quarters.

Tourists don't have to avoid the Jewish Quarter, but it's not as open as these other two quarters where people freely flow in and out. Women are expected to have their shoulders covered and to wear pants at least to the knee if they choose to enter the Western Wall women's section. We walk through the metal detector and security check point as we enter the Western Wall pavilion surrounded by Israeli soldiers guarding the perimeter. This is a holy place, always under heavy protection.

Two days ago, the pavilion had pulsed with bar mitzvah celebrations on the larger men's side. A high fence separates the men's and women's sections. One side was flanked by women stretching and straddling rickety benches and chairs to peak over the meshed fence to catch a glimpse of male family members celebrating on the other side.

Today is Shabbat. Quiet. Sherry and I sit on plastic chairs that line the side wall of the women's section, keenly aware of the contrast of Shabbat peace here and the violence at the Gaza Border. Tensions have increased during the past six months. When we purchased our trip insurance, it specified that acts of war would not be covered.

We gaze at the fence barrier that runs perpendicular to the Western Wall. Two sides of a wall that restrict access based on gender. Two passionate points of view. We live in a world of political divisions and have the southern-border wall back home that divides our country's citizens and restricts the access of refugees.

The wall is not crowded today, so it's easy to stand close and wedge our prayers into the crevasses between the bricks. Last night I wrote out prayers, one for each member of our immediate family, one more for our entire family, and one for Sherry. I know all the little slips of paper will be cleared out, but it feels good to slip my papers into a crevice, trusting they will travel to their rightful place. I place my hands on the warm bricks of the wall for a brief prayer of gratitude and hope. I stand and feel a soft vibration from the wall into my hands through my body.

"Do you know the historical reason for putting prayers between the stones of the Western Wall?" Sherry asks when I return to our chairs.

"No. Please tell me."

"I read that when King Solomon built the first Temple here in 826 BCE, he wanted it to be the heart of the Jewish nation. At the Temple's inauguration, he said, 'Hear the prayers that are said in this place.' So that's why we put our written prayers between the stones."

She continues, "I know we're related through Arnie, but you're becoming more like family to me. I would never have come to Israel if it hadn't been for you. When the Gaza violence erupted in May, I remember calling you, asking if we should postpone. You said, 'It will always be risky traveling to Israel. We just decide how much we want to do this.' And once you helped me decide, you helped me step out of my comfort zone in many other ways. I would never have walked into the Dead Sea if you hadn't gently encouraged me. You said, 'You will float and you will have an amazing time.' And I did."

"I was intimidated too, so it helped me to help you. I'm not always as brave as you think I am," I say, smiling. "And, I would never have gone to that fantastic light show in the Tower of David last night if you hadn't convinced me that we would love it. You point out little artistic things I don't notice. You encourage me to go off on my own with humor and without guilt. Just further proof that now we are family, friends, and awesome travel buddies."

We sit a while longer basking in the glow of the sun radiating off the Western Wall. Then we head back to the Jaffa Gate and sit down for a sip and snack. Three women walk up looking around for a place to sit. "Would you like to join us?" I ask them. "The table is small but we're heading out soon and then the table will be all yours."

"Oh yes!" They respond in chorus. "Thank you. We've been walking quite a while. Are you here with a tour?"

"We are. You too?"

"Yes!" one woman pipes up. "We have visited so many religious sites I never dreamed I'd see: Bethlehem, The Sea of Galilee, Nazareth. Have you visited those places yet?

"So, this must be a pilgrimage for you, walking in the footsteps of Jesus?" I say. "What a wonderful experience. Sherry and I are Jewish. Our tour includes many historic, archeological, and religious places. We see Israel through two different lenses. Different Israels for different beliefs," I say, smiling.

"You're right! And yet here we are, five pilgrims sitting together, enjoying this place, each other, and this moment," another woman offers.

We continue to sit and chat for a while, our tiny *ecumenical enclave* huddled around a small table sharing stories, discovering commonality. We ask someone to take pictures of us, vowing to treasure this sweet collegial gathering.

"Thank you for joining us. What wonderful timing!" I say as Sherry and I get up to go. "I'm glad we had the opportunity to share highlights of our tours and get to know each other. Best wishes. Safe travels."

And in a chorus, they say, "Shalom!"

The next days are filled with more excursions to surrounding areas, returning each night to our home base in Jerusalem. At one stop, Sherry and I stroll along the trails of the Qumran Caves where the Dead Sea Scrolls were stored, preserved, and then later discovered by Bedouin shepherds. The trail is wide. We can walk side by side, then stand and look up at the golden cliffs pocked with cave openings.

The guide stops. We stop. We wait. Then he pauses as if waiting for a drum roll and dramatically calls out, "Turn around. Look back. You are standing very close to Cave Number 4! This is the place where almost all the scrolls were discovered." We had already toured the museum that houses some of the scrolls. That was interesting. But standing at the site where they were stored and discovered is real and riveting.

A few days later we head south to Eilat. Tomorrow is a bonus relaxation day by the Red Sea for most. Sherry and I and six others from our group opted to use this free day to travel to Jordan and tour Petra. Early the next morning, we merge with another group of 18 tourists to travel to another different country, another world. First, we enter the Israeli check point to get our exit visas. Then we walk through fifty yards of *no man's land* until we enter the Jordan check point to obtain our entrance visas. Even though the two countries have been at peace since 1994, it's a bit unsettling to walk through this barren area between the two countries. Exciting too. Like being in a movie.

Our young loquacious tour guide, Daniel, greets us and explains we'll travel for almost two hours on the bus. "You are safe," he says. "We are safe. Our countries have signed a peace accord. Relax and enjoy this beautiful day." We head out and he happily describes places of interest, like the valley where they filmed *The Martian*, as we motor through the vast red rock landscape. Soon we arrive at Petra, also known as the Rose City, the ancient capital of the Nabataean Empire with its intricate carvings sculpted into red sandstone cliffs. We enter As Siq and walk through a steep narrow canyon that is almost dark as we look up, craning our necks until we finally see a thin sliver of bright blue sky framed by red rock.

The high walls radiate the racket of speeding donkey carts carrying tourists down the path. The narrow space is choked with activity. I find myself thinking, *This is nothing like the quiet tourist experience at Machu Picchu.* Then I catch myself. *Of course, not every place is going to be the same.* But still, this is very different. Vendors shout. Children run up begging us to buy. Daniel asks us not to purchase anything from them. "We have many groups working hard to reduce the disruption and distraction of this child labor. You will have the opportunity to purchase beautiful gifts made by artisans later in the tour. I understand you feel sorry and want to help them, but there are better ways to help."

At one of our rest stops, I ask Daniel, "Will we go all the way to the Monastery today? I'd love to climb the steps and tour that site."

Daniel shakes his head. "No, I'm sorry. This is an older group and we're going slow, so we won't have enough time to go all the way to the end and still stop for lunch and drive back to the border." He pauses. "So, you are curious and you like climbing stairs? Let me think of some other option for you."

"Oh, no no, Daniel. I just wanted to know. This is an amazing tour. I'm seeing more things than I ever dreamed of. I just wanted to understand how far we go."

We keep walking through the red-walled wonderland of ancient history and artistic excellence. The high walls are filled with intricate temple facades. There is even a theatre still remarkably intact carved into the side of the mountain.

We stop to rest, hydrate, and snack in the shade of a comfortable ramada. Sherry plays with a little kitten. I look around knowing this is our turn-around spot, hoping I can return sometime to explore the remaining sites.

Just as I look across the road and see a long flight of steps leading up to four structures carved high on a hill crest, Daniel asks for our attention. "We will stop here for about 20 minutes and then turn around and head back. Please make sure you drink enough. It will get hotter now with the sun straight overhead."

He pauses. "Now if any of you are interested in doing a little more exploring, you can cut your break short and climb up those stairs up to the Royal Tombs," he points across the street. "If you leave right now, you will have time to climb, explore, and then walk just a little faster to join us at the end. Is anybody interested in doing this?" He looks straight at me.

You are kidding me. Can this possibly be happening again? Am I being given another opportunity? This is too cool! I raise my hand along with two other couples. Daniel grins. "Okay! Go ahead, enjoy, and don't rush. You will have the time to climb, explore, and get back to meet us at the end."

"Bye, go have fun again," laughs Sherry. "See you later."

The five of us head across the path and start climbing steps carved into the mountain. My balance isn't great, so I walk close to the wall, touching it for support. One couple races ahead. The other couple, Jack and Sophie, walk up with me. We climb, chat, get to know each other. On the tight turns, Jack stands on the outside and lends his arm to Sophie so she can safely turn, then waits to do the same for me.

In the short time it takes to get up to the Palace Tomb we strangers manage to create that kind of sweet connection that tends to happen when a little trail magic seeps in. We take pictures of each other. Share our awe and pride that we ventured out and up those steps.

I walk through the door of the Palace Tomb and gasp. I've stepped into what looks like a large conference room surrounded by alcoved arches around all three sides. They are fenced off but still easy to get close enough to see intricate carvings and crannies. "Sandi, look up!" Sophie calls out.

The ceiling is covered with swirls of colored sand, a beautiful natural design, created by nature's paintbrush. "Thank you, Sophie! Breathtaking."

We can't linger. We take a few more pictures and then head back down the steps. I hold the wall and lean on Jack's arm on the turns. We head back out of As Siq at a steady pace, elated, laughing, congratulating ourselves. We reach the entrance just as the rest of the group is sitting down on the bleachers getting ready to wait for us. "I knew you'd make it!" yells Daniel, smiling, looking delighted. "We just finished our break, so let's head out."

"Sherry, how long did you have to wait?" I ask.

"We didn't! We got here about 15 minutes ago. Daniel gave us a short restroom and shopping break. We just sat down. Your timing was perfect."

Of course, it was. And this was another small unscripted,

unanticipated moment to remember and cherish.

Then we're back on the bus for our trip south to the border. "We made the right choice to include Petra on our trip," Sherry says, as we walk through no man's land together.

The next day we travel north back to Tel Aviv on the final day of our tour, still stopping and touring sites along the way.

We continue our drive passing by artillery, tanks, and walls and fences. While Mali explains the needs and benefits, I'm again acutely aware there are two sides to these barriers and many sides to the story.

A few hours later, we reach Tel Aviv for our flight home early the next morning.

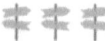

It's almost like I have been on one big trip since I retired. Venturing outside the country. Stepping way outside my comfort zone. I knew these experiences would change me. I had no idea of the extent. This is just my fourth trip out of North America, yet I feel like a world traveler in terms of lessons, experiences, moments, memories, and personal growth.

"It never hurts to ask" became my new travel mantra. Mali was delighted to give me Beit She'an in exchange for the Masada Snake Path. Daniel provided the climb up to the Royal Tombs in exchange for the Monastery steps. I more fully embraced the power of asking and accepting help, how it benefits the giver and receiver. I'm sure this lesson will continue to offer significant benefits as I keep exploring new places and climbing steps that will take me to brand new heights.

CHAPTER 8
Climbing High - Again

It's Thursday afternoon, January 2019. I've been retired for five years. And here I am, standing at the base of the lighthouse in the middle of the historic St. Augustine Light Station campus at the start of my weekly 2.5-hour volunteer shift. My official role as a member of the lighthouse team is to greet visitors, ensure they are safe, and answer their questions.

This afternoon is cool and quiet, no school or big tour groups, just a few guests. I will have more than enough time to perform the other fun functions I've added to my role over the past few years, those of motivator, photographer, and exerciser.

I chat with Linda, the 78-year-old volunteer I have relieved since I started volunteering here four years ago. Linda serves as the historian and usually follows up her standard greeting to guests with a brief history lesson. "Be sure to check out the two museums as you enter the lighthouse. On one side of the hallway is the keeper's office; on the other side is the fuel room where the lighthouse keepers used to store and heat the fuel. They would have to carry the processed fuel up the steps in 30-pound containers to power the light in the days before electricity."

We're each wearing our uniform of royal-blue polo shirts and volunteer name tags. Linda wears khaki pants. I wear khaki Bermuda Shorts because it's more comfortable to climb up and down the lighthouse in them. And my knee-replacement surgery scars encourage many lighthouse guests. "You can climb to the top of the lighthouse with those knees? Well, if you can do it, so can I."

Just then a man and woman walk into the patio, pushing up their sleeves to show me their entrance wristbands. The woman gazes up at the looming lighthouse and then at me. She looks nervous. Her husband looks excited.

"Welcome to the Saint Augustine Light Station! Are you going to climb? Is this your first lighthouse?"

"Yes and yes," she replies. "But now I'm not so sure. It's been on my bucket list so long. I really want to climb up to the top, but I had no idea it would be this tall."

"It's definitely daunting." I need her to know how much I respect her anxiety and fear. "I'm comfortable climbing this lighthouse, but I'm absolutely terrified to drive over certain bridges even though they're not that scary to most folks. We each have our own real fears."

She cocks her head and gives me a soft smile, so I continue, "It's one thing to look at a lighthouse from the distance. It's entirely different when you get close and look all the way up to the 165-foot top. I won't try to convince you not to be scared, but I'd like to give you some information that might help you decide what you want to do. Okay?"

"Okay." Her shoulders relax.

"First, you're exactly right. It's tall. This is the second tallest lighthouse in Florida. From here at the base up to the red observation deck you will climb 219 steps. That's 14 stories. And you'll stand on a platform 140-feet high. It's a monumental accomplishment."

She stands and listens. I continue, "When you step out on the deck you will feel like you're standing on top of the world, able to see 20 miles in every direction, each view with its own unique beauty."

"When I first started to volunteer here, my focus was always on getting to the top. I was frustrated that I'd had to stop at each landing to catch my breath. Soon, I learned that the journey up that incredible circular staircase is just as delightful as seeing those vast views at the top. Climbing one step at a time, stopping, and resting on each of the eight broad landings is exhilarating. Continuing to ascend until you step out on the red platform is— breath-taking."

She hasn't moved. Still listening. I keep talking. "One of the best things about this lighthouse is that it has railings on both sides of the steps all the way up. I always use them. They help me feel safe and secure. It is also very user-friendly with deep steps you can put your whole foot on. And here is the best news of all: the staircase is wide enough so people can comfortably pass each other in either direction. You can turn around at any time."

"Really?" she says. "Do you mean if I start up and decide I want to stop, I can just turn around and go down?"

"Absolutely! This is *your* climb. You take this lighthouse journey as far as you want. You can turn around at any point. Many climbers opt to stop at one of the eight landings, turn around, and climb back down. And you picked the perfect day. It's cool, clear, and not at all crowded." She smiles.

I move in to close the deal, "How about this—would you consider climbing up to the second landing? There is a deep window where you can see the Atlantic Ocean. It's beautiful! You can even sit on the sill and enjoy the view while your husband climbs all the way to the top. What do you think?"

She laughs. "Okay, you sold me. I'll do it. I'll climb to the second landing." Her husband standing behind her unfurls a crinkly-eyed grin and gives me an enthusiastic thumbs-up.

They head into the lighthouse, both with big smiles. I'm smiling too. Encouraging visitors to take baby steps is one of my most favorite things to do. I can easily have this conversation multiple times during each of my shifts. Many visitors want to climb until they walk into the patio and look up, up, up. They need genuine understanding and respect. Occasionally a soft nudge. Some say no, and I don't push any further. But most say yes.

Here's the best part: most of the people I encourage to climb to the window on the second landing end up going all the way to the top! What a rush for them—and me.

I'm making a difference one person at a time. Helping someone achieve their dream is my dream come true. My lighthouse purpose.

And those who don't climb all the way to the top are delighted with their short climb up to the second landing. When they come down, they usually say something like, "I didn't go the whole way to the top, but I climbed up those lighthouse steps and got up to the first window and that's good enough for me."

"You bet. You climbed the St. Augustine Lighthouse and saw beauty from on high! Good for you!"

As I stand by the base during a brief lull, a brisk breeze whisks my thoughts back over the years and across the miles to Columbus, Ohio, 2013, just a few months before I retired. I was wrapping and packing up my career at Limited Brands.

Work had been a satisfying part of my life for almost 50 years. But I was ready to move on. It felt good to say goodbye with gratitude, knowing I had made a difference in a few big ways and many little ways.

In my various jobs throughout my working years, I had been a teacher, consultant, manager, student, most recently here a Human Resources VP of Learning and Development. Making a difference in those roles was satisfying, even exhilarating.

Also connecting. Learning from many. Inspiring others, especially since I had already become the *old woman* who happened to walk, hike, and climb a lot. Most colleagues described me as passionate. I loved what I did.

But most of my passion was dedicated to family. In fact, one recruiter told me early in my career, "If you apply even a fraction of your family commitment to your job, you will be incredibly successful." I was.

But when I retired, I wanted something different, a role and connections that would satisfy and complete me in a new way. It was time to start exploring.

One night I said to Arnie, "I wonder what inspiration, people, and purpose will replace what I gained from work. I know volunteering will fill some of that need."

"You mean you're going to do even more volunteering than you already do? We fix meals at the women's shelter, you crochet blankets, you create and send all those cards to people, many you don't even know."

"Most of that other stuff I already do at home while we watch TV. We'll still volunteer at shelters and food banks, but we don't do that on a regular basis. I need something more defined when I retire. I want to make a difference that I can see and feel on a regular basis. I had to work for an income, but also, I enjoyed work because it fueled my passion. I want that same feeling now that I'm retired and don't need the income."

Arnie shook his head, furled his brows, paused. "You've spent so many years working hard, rushing around trying to pack in all the things you love to do into every day. You're often frustrated and stressed that you don't have enough time to do it all. I'm just worried that you'll keep up that same pace after you retire. That you won't have time. That *we* won't have the time to simply be together."

I needed to stop, listen carefully, and understand what was concerning Arnie. Although he had held several engaging jobs throughout the years, his main career had always been caregiver and anchor even after the kids left home.

But things had changed recently. He had both hips and knees replaced. So did I. But I had emerged from my surgeries even stronger while Arnie's medical issues had increased. He had started to slow down, spending more time at home. I realized my retirement had to offer new opportunities for both of us.

"You're right. I *have* been too frantic too long," I reassured him. "We need our time together. I will slow down and finally capture that balance that has eluded me. I too want peace, time to simply sit and finish our conversations before rushing off to do something else."

Arnie's face relaxed. He started nodding, smiling. "Okay. Please take time to think about all those things you've wanted to do when you retire, like taking long walks in the morning, and even writing that book that has been banging around in your head all these years. I just don't want volunteering to take up so much of your time that you don't have time for us and those other dreams sitting on the back shelf."

"I agree. Just a few hours a week. I don't want this to turn into another job."

I pushed my volunteering quest to the back burner during the first year after retirement while we settled in and made new lifestyle decisions. Arnie had followed me around the country with my career. Now it was *his* turn to choose where we would live. He was done with cold and snow. Ready for warmth and water. So, we landed in Palm Coast, Florida, ten miles west of the Atlantic Ocean and just a few blocks away from the Intracoastal Waterway.

Most of our family was finally on the East Coast. Rachel, Rob, and our two older grandsons, Jonathan (named after his uncle), and Andrew, lived in Lexington Park, Maryland.

Jonathan and Lauren had divorced years ago, but we remained family. She is our daughter-in-law, mother of our two younger grandsons. We are her mother and father-in-law, grandparents to the boys. She and our two younger grandsons, Jonathan (nicknamed Flip to help us keep the three *Jonathans* in our family straight) and Sam lived in St. Augustine. Our son, Jonathan, at that time was on board the USS Nimitz, an aircraft carrier somewhere in the Pacific serving as a U.S. Navy Supply Officer.

I was prepared for the heat and humidity now that we were back in Florida, but just as I was surprised by the beauty in and around Orlando, I was stunned with the plethora of nature preserves, local parks, and walking/biking trails in northeastern Florida. There was even a linear trail in a forested area between a divided highway.

But I still missed the elevation changes. Even in Columbus I could climb the stairs at work, the long flights of steps at Hoover Dam, even in hospital stairwells when Arnie was a patient.

Arnie went searching and found a short set of steps close to home by the Highway 100 Bridge over the Intracoastal Waterway.

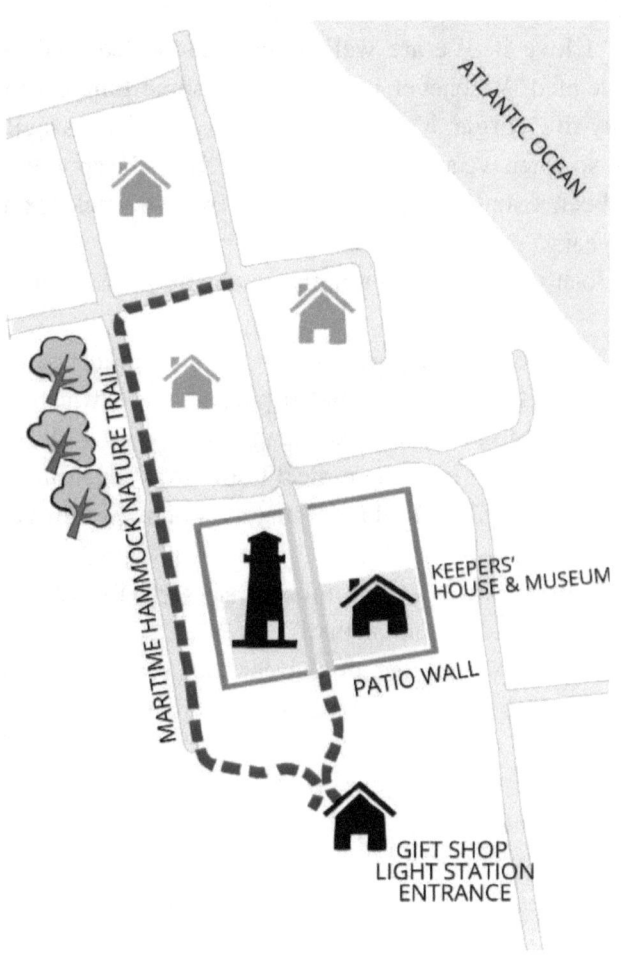

Then I remembered that one of the most beautiful lighthouses in Florida was right up Highway A1A just forty-five minutes north of Palm Coast in St. Augustine. It was not a mountain, but it was a great place to climb.

I started driving up to meet Lauren, Flip, and Sam so we could climb the lighthouse together. A seed was planted. *This might be a great place to volunteer.* It started to germinate on our next visit when I noticed a volunteer name tag on the person standing at the base. "Hi, Josh. How do you like volunteering here?"

"I love it. We are well trained, supported, and very much appreciated. Whenever I want to take some time off to visit my family in Georgia, it's no big deal. Each shift is assigned to paid staff, so when we aren't here, they just fill in the spot. It's all good. I've been volunteering here once or twice a week for more than five years."

Josh was right. I found my place, my purpose, and so much more.

My attention snapped back to the present just as two elderly men in baggy blue jeans, faded polo shirts, and iconic baseball caps walk into the courtyard engaged in a spirited discussion. As they get closer, I hear the typical tug-of-war regarding the climb. "I am not climbing! I told you that as soon as we drove up," says Mr. Reluctant.

"Yes, you are. You promised," says Mr. Pushy.

"When did I promise that?"

"When we got out of the car and saw that family at the entrance. You said, 'If they can do it, I can do it.'"

"Oh. Yeah. I forgot."

By this time, they're standing at the bottom of the stairs looking at me, reading my name tag. "Let's ask Sandi what she thinks."

Mr. Reluctant rolls his eyes. "Well of course she's going to agree with you. Right, Sandi?"

"Maybe, but before I answer your question, I'd like to thank you both for your service," acknowledging their Vietnam Veteran caps.

They pause, take a breath, then relax. "Thank you. My name is Rob. I don't want to climb even though I said I would. And my pushy partner's name is Roy. Nice to meet you, Sandi."

"Nice to meet you. Now let me give you a little information that might help you feel more comfortable about climbing."

Rob holds up his hand. "Say no more. I just need to know one thing, Sandi." He cocks his head and grins. "Do you ever climb the whole 219 steps to the top? Because if you climb it, I'll climb it." Now he's starting to flirt. (It happens. Must be the uniform).

I smile and respond, "Yes, I do. Every week I climb up the tower at least once before my shift, and sometimes again when my shift ends."

Rob's shoulders sag for a moment. "So you climb all 219 steps?" He looks at the steps leading into the lighthouse, cranes his neck up, sighs, then nods. "Okay, a deal is a deal. I'll go ahead and climb this tower with old Roy here."

They climb to the top of the concrete stairs leading to the entrance hallway. I hold up my hand, "Wait, here's the best news of all. You've already climbed 5 steps. You only have 214 steps left!"

They hoot and howl, their laughter echoing through the short hall as they advance to the circular staircase. A moment later the reluctant wife and encouraging husband walk down the steps.

"Guess what, Sandi!" exclaims the wife. "I got to the second landing and after resting for a few minutes and enjoying the view, I decided to climb a few more landings. I ended up climbing all the way to the top! I would never have climbed today if you hadn't encouraged me. I checked something off my bucket list because of you. Thank you!"

She hugs me. Her husband can't stop grinning. Neither can I. We stand, savor this moment. We all succeeded. Then I offer, "I'd love to take a picture of you in front of the lighthouse so you can always remember this milestone. Do you have a phone?"

"Oh yes." The husband whips out his phone and hands it to me.

"Please follow me," I say as I lead them down the walk from the lighthouse to the lighthouse keepers' house. They look confused as we walk away from the lighthouse.

"Trust me. Look at me. And prepare to be amazed." I scroll to *panorama,* turn the phone sideways and start moving the phone up, up, up to the top of the lighthouse. When I show them the photo of the two of them with the entire lighthouse in the background, they are amazed. Just as I knew they would be.

They gasp and gush, "This is our best picture ever! We will always have this picture to remember the lighthouse and you. Thanks again, Sandi."

A few other visitors are looking on and start lining up for me to take their pictures too. This is *so* much fun, taking the perfect family picture with the entire length of the lighthouse in the background. I take the picture, show it to them, humbly pause for the *ooohhs* and *aaahhs.* Their smiles are contagious. Their delight palpable. Little things like perfect family pictures help create a magical experience for our lighthouse guests.

While I'm busy taking pictures, Rob and Roy come out of the lighthouse, head out of the patio, and give me two thumbs up. Rob winks at me. Of course.

A little boy comes tearing into the courtyard. "Jamie, wait up! You can't go in there alone. Freeze!" He screeches to a halt, grins, and waves at me. His mom rushes in, followed by his dad, laughing.

They walk up to the lighthouse entrance, all three chattering, rolling up their sleeves to show me their wristbands. Jamie walks up to me and sticks his arm out. "See my band? The lady inside measured me and I'm finally tall enough to climb the lighthouse!"

Reaching a height of 44 inches is a major milestone. "I can

see why you're so excited. Congratulations! How old are you?"

"I'm five." He holds up his hand, fingers spread wide. His smile is even wider.

"Wow! You are climbing a lighthouse at five? Did you know some people don't climb until they are much older?"

"I know! My dad has never climbed a lighthouse before, so this will be his first time too." I look at Dad. His eyes are still happy, but his grin has morphed into a slight grimace.

I bend down to look Jamie in the eye just as he's getting ready to tear up the stairs. I must calm him down so he will be safe, and his parents can relax a bit. "You have a big job today taking care of your dad. All you have to do is hold onto the railing and go slowly and he will be fine. Okay?"

"Okay!"

Both parents whisper "Thank you," then turn to climb the stairs.

My shift starts to wind down. Dorothy, a young staff member, walks over. She knows about my stair climbing and had told me she wants to be as active as I am when she is in her 70s. I had told her how I got started with the Grand Canyon R2R2R and she exclaimed, "I've heard of that! That's on my bucket list. Something I want to do. It's hard to believe you kept going after three *DNF's*. Who does that?"

I laughed, "Lots of people. The ones who refuse to give up."

She shook her head. "Well, I want to hike within the next few years, so all I need is a friend who will do it with me. You are such an inspiration, the way you climb the stairs and participate in events. Thank you."

"You're welcome. Good for you. It might be harder to train in Florida, but thank goodness you have ready access to the lighthouse."

Just as Dorothy walks away, Jamie bounces down the stairs and runs over to me. "I did it, Miss Sandi! I climbed all the way to the top and so did my dad!"

When his mom and dad join him, clearly delighted and relieved, I say, "I'd love to take a picture of you in front of the lighthouse so you can always remember today. Do you have a phone?"

The sun moves behind the lighthouse as the day progresses. "Hi, Sandi, ready to head home for today?" says John, the staff employee who will cover the closing shift.

"I didn't have time to do my five climbs before my shift, so I'm going to do them now. It's just three more weeks before the American Lung Association Fight for Air stair climb I told you about, so I need to get in as much training as I can."

"That stair climb is such a neat event. I have lived here so many years and can't believe I never heard of it before you started volunteering here. I might recruit a few friends and do it next year," says John. "I could use a bit of stair climbing to stay in shape like you do."

I start my climb, gripping the railing of that sturdy staircase and gradually glide up the steps in a slow and steady pace. I no longer need to stop and catch my breath, surprised at how easy this climb has become after my years of volunteering and recent weeks of training. I step up and celebrate the power of practice.

I reach the top and take a quick peak into the small room that holds the first order Fresnel lens with its 370 individual prisms and 3 bullseyes. For a moment I ponder the magic of this lens that can radiate beams of light 30+ miles from a 1000-watt light bulb. One light source that illuminates the sky every night. It reminds me of small gestures that can spread joy, rippling, replicating, brightening lives.

I step out at the bright red platform that encircles the tower, take a brief look around, wave at Jay, the tower volunteer. "See you for four more climbs."

He laughs, "Go for it! Great time to get your five climbs in this week."

I descend the 200+ steps, turn around at the bottom of the

circular staircase, and start my second climb, a little faster this time but never too fast, just smooth, steady, and safe.

After my five climbs, I wave goodbye to John and head out of the patio through the gift shop and out to the parking lot.

I sit in my car for a few minutes and reflect on how well lighthouse volunteering has fit into my retired life. I love the rewarding reciprocity of interacting with lighthouse guests as I inform, influence, and sometimes even inspire them. Volunteering at the lighthouse provides everything I want, at least for now. It's outside, athletic, flexible, engaging. I make a difference. I'm connected to staff members. I support a worthy organization.

My investment of time at the lighthouse is small compared to its bountiful return. I spend 1.5 hours driving round trip to St. Augustine and 2.5 hours on my shift. I usually add an extra hour to climb the lighthouse and walk around the nature preserve. The total time I normally spend each week is 5 hours, and that includes an hour of my own exercise time!

Retirement granted me the gift of more time and greater control over my life. My life expanded. Arnie and I have all the time we want to sit and chat, actually finishing our conversations. We are balanced; not bored. Life is full; not frenzied. We are members of a spiritual community. We contribute. We donate time, serving meals to the homeless. We've even started cooking our meals together. We walk almost every day. Connecting with neighbors. Petting their dogs. We have sweet and unique relationships with each member of our family. He has his activities closer to home. I have mine more widespread.

It's a little after 4:00. The sun is moseying west as I drive out of the lighthouse parking lot and turn left on A1A heading south to Palm Coast. I approach one of my favorite sections, a narrow strip of land with whitecaps and waves of the Atlantic Ocean on my left and the calm, lazy Intracoastal Waterway on my right.

I enter a meditative space. Being a St. Augustine Lighthouse volunteer is now part of my identity, even to my family. Flip asked if I was still volunteering at the lighthouse in his interview for a class project last week. When I said yes, he smiled, "Oh good!" Some people don't know my name, but they know I volunteer and climb the lighthouse each week.

I glance at the panorama of blue skies caressing the ocean migrating over to the nascent glow of the setting sun kissing the ICW. It reminds me of a big, beautiful 1000-piece jigsaw puzzle and how frustrating it can be when you're almost finished and there are still a few pieces missing. It doesn't matter that that you have most pieces in place.

At first my life seemed to contain the necessary facets of successful retirement. Necessary but not sufficient. My retirement was missing something, a new sense of purpose. So, I kept looking and finally found those final missing pieces at the St Augustine Lighthouse.

My picture is complete. At least for now.

CHAPTER 9
Stepping Up

Way back in 2004, during my annual physical, I told Dr. Liskow, "I've started having severe pain in my right hip, especially after I walk four or five miles. I even canceled plans to fly down to Orlando to walk another Walt Disney World Marathon with my brother. I hate to be a wimp, but I wonder if I should take some pain relievers."

Dr. Liskow pressed my leg, telling me to push and pull. "Your legs are strong," he remarked. "Did you fall? Any injuries?"

"No, it's just sore after I walk longer distances," I replied.

"Well, before we change any medication, let's get some X-rays," he suggested.

A few weeks later his nurse called. "Sandi, you have severe arthritis in your right hip. Dr. Liskow wants you to see an orthopedist as soon as possible."

I went for my appointment, more curious than worried. Then, I got mad.

I am at my best with Arnie. I can also be at my worst.

I came home, storming, raging. "I am getting a second opinion. You won't believe that doctor's diagnosis! He said my hip was so deteriorated he didn't even know how I was still able to walk. And then he had the nerve to tell me I need hip-replacement surgery! He's just knife happy. He's looking at me like I'm some feeble old lady. He didn't even suggest physical therapy." I finally stopped to take a breath.

Long pause. Arnie waited for me to calm down.

"Do you want me to do some research on another doctor?" Arnie offered.

"No!" I said, in determined denial. "I'll just use more Biofreeze and get a few more massages. It can't possibly be as bad as he said."

Arnie had two artificial knees and infinitely more perspective. "Did he show you the X-ray?" he quietly asked.

"Yes. It looked bad, but there's no way I'm having my hip replaced," I said adamantly. "I am too young. I've heard your range of motion gets totally destroyed. I'll never be able to hike again. I'd rather live in pain. I can manage."

I was just 60 years old and active, not a couch potato, and not a runner or a jumper. *How could this happen to me?* I held off for another year until my joint was so abscessed and immobile, I could barely walk, sit, or sleep. (I sure showed that orthopedist!)

I had the surgery on my right hip in April 2005, knowing my other joints were also breaking down. I learned some valuable lessons that helped me navigate the rest of my surgery years. First, I did not wait so long for the other three replacements. As soon as my quality of life began to suffer, I started the process. Second, I switched surgeons after my first surgery. Making this change was daunting, but I wanted one who was more proactive in terms of pre- and post-rehab.

Many people tell me, "It's so impressive that you do so much climbing, hiking, and walking with four artificial joints." But my artificial joints are my friends. I can't imagine doing what I do without them. I'm lucky. I'm fortunate.

My mother struggled with arthritis and could barely walk by the time she was my age because her knees hurt so much. Joint replacement was not nearly as prevalent 25 years ago. I'm thankful for my metal joints! In fact, my four joint-replacement surgeries have also helped me develop some major *resilience* muscles as I went from hiking and walking at least 15-25 miles a week to hobbling 100 yards to the mailbox with a walker after each surgery.

I'm used to starting over at zero. I've had lots of practice.

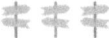

And now it's February 2019. Natalie and I catch our breath as we relax by a portable barre during break in our ballet exercise class. With effervescent chatter and laughter in the background, we congratulate ourselves on our 75th birthdays. She just celebrated hers. Mine is in two weeks.

"This class is so cool. It feels like recess, back when we were kids. This is even more fun," I say.

Natalie agrees. "Right. We are healthy and active, and don't have too much wrong with us. It's good."

Natalie is tall like me. And very slender, not like me. She's the same weight she was when she got married as she loves telling everyone. I feel a twinge of envy when I hear this. Though I'm sort of slender now, I yo-yo'd through many years of gains and losses. Filmmaker and author Nora Ephron felt bad about her neck. My neck is okay. But I feel bad about my batwing upper arms and lumpy thighs. My knees are pudgy. Calves aren't too bad. My body shape is a mixed bag. But it works well, and I can walk long and far. Good enough.

My hair started turning grey when I was in my teens. I let it have its way with its color except for that one time in high school when I tried to dye it using red Jell-O. (Thankfully, it washed out quickly). Since then, I've kept it simple. I adopted an even easier style when I turned 65 and was planning to spend three nights at Phantom Ranch at the bottom of the Grand Canyon with my friend Carole. No way was I going to pack a hair dryer down the Bright Angel Trail! My current *wash and wear* style looks good enough, short, slightly wavy, and gradually getting whiter. I like my hair.

I look around the room at the 30 women standing by the

portable ballet barres. At least ten of us are in our seventies, maybe 15 or so in their sixties, a few youngsters in their late fifties, and just one woman in her eighties. Some have missed classes due to illness or injuries. Many of those injuries were caused by falling. Some women are cancer survivors. Most have other issues: arthritis, asthma, and the usual aches and pains associated with aging. We are fortunate and grateful, determined to be fit and stay active. This room filled with strong women is a *no excuse zone.*

As Natalie and I walk out at the end of the session, she says, "We need this class. We have to keep maintaining our health or we will start to break down." She throws her arm over my shoulders. "If we keep doing this, we don't really have to worry about getting too old until we're 80. I think that's when the trouble starts."

She waves goodbye and heads to her car. Natalie's words make me feel good at first, but that warning about 80 keeps rattling around in my head.

I walk home, taking the longer two-mile route. Most days I take a short nap after lunch. But not on my lighthouse day. Sometimes I time-box activities, but never my time with Arnie. We sit and catch up on our morning as he takes a break from working out on his recumbent stepper machine. I finish the laundry, eat lunch, shower, and change clothes. Then head out early so I can do my final five training climbs for the American Lung Association Stair Climb before my shift starts.

I walk out to the car and say my *car prayer*, something I had started a few years ago when we moved to Florida. My belief in a supreme being is fluid. My belief in the power of prayer is rock solid. I say my please and thank you prayers each morning and evening, and recently added this prayer when we started driving on I-95, a treacherous stretch of Florida highway. "Please keep us safe. And let it be a good drive for all. Amen."

Once I'm on A1A, I allow my mind to tackle some tough questions I've been wrestling with. At times, turning 75 is a bigger deal than I thought it would be. I'm one step closer to 80. Even closer to 79, the age my mom died. She had been incredibly active, but in her 70s she stopped her exercise walking due to her sore knees. She started putting on weight. I thought she'd live well into her 80s like my grandmother. I did not expect her to die so young. I don't think she did either.

Since age 45 when the R2R2R changed my life, I started losing weight to walk, not the other way around. I still yo-yoed, but I was always especially diligent before a big event, saying to myself, "Just remember how much easier it will be for you to climb, walk, and especially hike. Every step you take will be 5-10 pounds lighter."

I stopped eating meat except fish last year, so that's made it much easier to manage my weight and my digestion system.

I'm healthy. I'm lucky. I have not had cancer except several basal cell lesions on my face that have been removed using Mohs surgery. These surgeries left a few scattered scars on my face, which is ironic since these basal cell issues were caused by the X-ray treatments that were used back in the day to treat my serious, scarring teenage acne.

My bouts with bursitis and sciatica have given me an increased level of compassion for those who suffer from debilitating and persistent nerve pain. My atrial fib is controlled with meds and my capable cardiologist, Dr. Dinesh Pubbi, who listens to my heart and my travel stories. My cataracts were removed last year, so my eyes are fine too.

None of that stuff had been embarrassing or hard to discuss, but then I encountered urinary incontinence. I had to urinate—often—seemed like all the time. My latest in a long *stream* of medications were no longer working. So, last year my primary care physician referred me to a urologist, Dr. Julie Schneider, who provided understanding and options. At first, I tried a Botox treatment because it seemed less invasive, but I found out later it caused other issues.

After that didn't work, I opted for inter-stem implant surgery, which was scheduled the next month after a viability test. This implant is like a pacemaker for my bladder and could reduce my visits to the bathroom by almost 50%.

At first it was hard for me to share my urge-incontinence issues with friends, but now I am more comfortable trading stories since many have similar issues. And I have refused to let it stop me from any events, trips, or treks. There's a good reason for all those thick panty pad brands.

So, 75 is pretty good. But Natalie may be right about trouble starting at 80 even though I had convinced myself to look forward to the next decade with anticipation. The only 80-year-old in our class is amazing: strong, slender, limber, and active. But where are the other women in their 80s? What happened to others as they moved through their 70s? Where did they go? Are they staying home? Why?

Our Tai Chi class is taught by an incredible gentleman, Wil Hessert, known as "The General." Wil is 78 and a retired USAF Major General. He served 42 years in the Armed Forces. He embraced a new practice and purpose after his retirement from the military, continuing his service in a very different way. Wil is a passionate, compassionate, disciplined, and dedicated instructor who imparts his Tai Chi routines along with his own healing stories as we stand, breathe, balance, and meditate in his weekly classes. "Relax, relax, relax," he softly murmurs as we move through our postures and poses.

There are three men and four women in my class who are in their 80s. It is fun being with some *real* seniors, hearing their stories, giving me hope. I love how they manage to work their age into each conversation. I say good morning to Fred, and he quickly reminds me, "You know Rob is turning 83 next month and I'm going to be 87!"

When we get short breaks to grab water and chat with others, the ambient noise usually increases to a level that requires Wil to bang the gong a couple of times to let us know when break time is over.

Joan is one of my favorite break partners. She's a bit shorter than I am, fit and sturdy with short, wavy, grey hair. She doesn't wear any makeup. Her naturally bright and kind eyes dominate her softly wrinkled face. She and I chat for a few minutes. I ask my usual question, "So, Joan, have you always been this active?"

"I'm 84 almost 85," she says. "I used to ride my bike and walk a lot like you. I don't walk as much anymore but I still get out when I can. And of course, I come to Tai Chi every week. And I watch what I eat."

I smile. "You are my inspiration. You give me hope that if I keep walking, watch what I eat, and stay active, I can be like you at your age."

"Thank you, Sandi! You're much younger than I but you still inspire me to get out and walk as much as possible. Especially when you tell me your lighthouse and Grand Canyon stories. We're good for each other."

Another Tai Chi colleague is also fit at 85. Soon to be 86, he reminds me. Art is a Palm Coast historian who has written several books on the history of this area. We're chatting during another break, and he says quietly, "Sandi, I recently learned I have Alzheimer's. So, while I can still remember historical facts, there will be a day I may not remember your name. But when I see you, I will always remember your zest for life, your smile, your passion, your commitment to the lighthouse, and your interest in everyone else in our class."

We look at each other. Everything else fades into the background. I take a deep breath. "I don't want you to worry about forgetting my name. From now on as soon as I see you, I'll say, 'Hi, Art, I'm Sandi. Good to see you.' Is that a deal?"

Art smiles and nods. "It's a deal."

We stand together a few more moments, alone in our quiet space.

Then the gong sounds.

Ballet exercise is like home room and recess in an all-girls school with on-going chatter throughout the entire class. We are led by our capable and amazing instructor, Terry Burde, who volunteers her time to lead this class and many others.

During one of our breaks, I chat with an attractive strong woman well into her 80s. "You are so fit. Have you always been this active and healthy?"

"Oh, hell no," she exclaims. "I smoked all through my 50s; I was a couch potato and I suffered from emphysema. And then out of the blue someone asked me if I wanted to run a 10K with her. I did and placed first in my age group. I got hooked. Even ran some half marathons. I don't do events anymore, but I take at least three exercise classes each week. And when you invited our whole class for that BYO lunch and presentation at the St Augustine Lighthouse, I climbed all the way to the top!"

One day, I'm leaving class with Nancy Brandon, also in her mid-seventies. "You are important for us," she says. "You are our role model for coming to class with artificial joints. Before you started, many other women stopped coming after they had joint-replacement surgery. They gave up. But now we see you with all four joints, lifting your legs up on the barre, doing it all, and even climbing the lighthouse every week. You have taught us that joint-replacement surgery is no reason to quit staying active and fit."

Tai Chi and ballet exercise classes enhance my strength, balance, and flexibility. The collective caring warms my heart and fills my soul. I am healthier in body and mind because I take these classes.

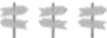

I arrive early at the lighthouse, so I have ample time to climb my five loops before starting my shift. I wave to Linda and start climbing the stairs thinking, *All I need to think about today is picturing myself on the Bank of America stairs on Saturday. Just focus on your formula: One lighthouse climb of 200+ steps equals 10 stories.* The climb is 713 steps 36 stories. So, 36 stories equal 3.5 lighthouse climbs. Got it. I loved creating my own training formulas.

I finish my five loops in 35 minutes and still have 30 minutes before my shift begins. Just then Barb Holland walks over. She is my long-time staff back-up and facilitator of the two luncheon groups I had sponsored earlier that year. One for my ballet exercise class and the other for The Compassionate Women of St. Augustine. She captivated both audiences with her "Women of the Lighthouse" stories, especially the one where Junior Service League members stood in front of the bulldozers stopping the destruction of the lightkeepers' house. "Hey, Sandi, I know you've told me this before, but what exactly are you doing on Saturday?"

I love telling people about the Fight for Air stair climb. I started participating in this event in Columbus in 2013, four months after my second knee-replacement surgery. Stacy, a young woman who saw me climbing up and down the stairs at work told me about the stair climb and asked me if I would join her little Limited Brands team. I agreed and then recruited Miriam Siegfried from our temple book club. She and I started training together on the weekends and began a new climbing friendship that has spanned the years. The first year we moved to Florida, I did both climbs—one in Columbus and one here in Jacksonville. Miriam still participates every year in Columbus, climbing fast and raising record-setting donations. And I am getting ready for my eighth ALA climb.

I explain to Barb, "Fight for Air is one of those few events that raises money and increases awareness in a physical, tangible way. We participants literally fight for air as we climb the steps, getting a small sense of what it means to struggle as we climb higher and higher, gasping for air, fighting for each breath as we push ourselves to the top. Of course, we *choose* to fight for air. The many who suffer from lung disease have no choice. We climb for them."

Barb says. "It sounds like a perfect event for those of us who spend time at the lighthouse. I may try it next year."

Barb, Linda, and I split up as I turn to greet a family getting ready to climb. "Welcome to the St Augustine Lighthouse. You have picked a great day to climb…"

After my shift, I drive home thinking mainly about Saturday's climb. It's the perfect event to kick off my year-long 75th birthday celebration.

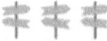

After all my training and experience, I still have trouble sleeping Friday night, and wake up at 3:00 Saturday morning with a nervous stomach. Frustrating, but not surprising. Just part of my usual pre-event process. The pain before the gain.

The boys spent Friday night with Jonathan, so I drive up to Lauren's house and we ride to the Bank of America building together. "Thank you so much for doing this with me every year, Lauren. And for getting Flip involved a few years ago. I think this is our fifth anniversary."

"Oh, of course!" Lauren laughs. "I remember how you gradually enticed and recruited me, sealing the deal when you listed all the benefits of supporting the American Lung Association in such a tangible way. And we trained at the lighthouse that first year Flip joined us. I have dropped the ball on my training these past couple of years. But I still love it, especially that we three do it together. It's our thing. And a nice way to make a difference."

We walk into the Bank of America. I feel like I'm ready to jump out of my skin. *C'mon, Sandi, get a grip. It will take less than 15 minutes*!

Jonathan and the boys are waiting for us in the crowded noisy lobby. "Hi, Mom, you ready to go?" Jonathan asks as Flip and Sam come over to hug me.

"I am, but I'm still crazy nervous," I say, shaking my head.

"It will all be over soon, right? And you'll do fine, right? You know you always do, Mom. Let's stand by the poster and I'll get someone to take our picture."

We get our picture taken. Lauren and I walk to the bathroom. There's a long line. "Looks like we're not the only ones who are a little hyper," Lauren laughs.

Lauren, Flip, and I get in line. Jonathan and Sam stand to the side holding our stuff, waiting near the stairwell entrance so they can cheer and snap some photos of our start. There are about 20 people ahead of us. We can see the bright lights and hear the chant, "One, two, three, go!" Loud cheers. Another twenty seconds, "One, two, three, go!"

"Flip can go first this time since he's the fastest. I'll go and then you, okay, Sandi?" Lauren says. I nod, take another sip of water, and hand the bottle to Jonathan.

Flip steps up to the line. The volunteer puts her hand on his shoulder, smiles at him. "Ready to go?" Flip nods. It's his third climb. He knows the drill. "One, two, three, go." He runs across the timing pad, into the door and disappears into the stairwell.

Lauren's turn. Then mine. I start my Apple watch, take a deep breath, smile at Jonathan and Sam. I walk over the timing pad into the stairwell and brace myself for the first few moments of claustrophobia in the quiet dead-space of the fire-escape stairs. I climb, calm my breathing, and quietly review my strategy. "Start slow. Gradually increase speed until the 32nd floor. Then pour it on, push my legs and fight for air as I race to floor 36."

It's still. Silent. I climb, slowly, gripping the rails, listening carefully so I can quickly step aside when I hear someone barreling up the stairs behind me. The stairs reverberate. Two runners pass in quick succession, then a third climber bounces by taking two steps at a time.

Quiet again. Just the soft slap of my shoes on the stairs. I climb, turn at the landings, ignore the floor numbers, and focus on my breathing: *steady, strong, steady.* I know I'm getting close to the 10th floor when I hear volunteers cheer as they hand out little cups of water. "Good job, keep going, you're looking great!"

10th floor. One lighthouse. I congratulate myself. "Good job Sandi, just two and a half more lighthouses to go." I see one person who had passed me earlier hugging the landing wall gasping, gulping a second cup of water. I speed up a bit but keep a steady pace, so I don't have to stop to catch my breath.

20th floor. Two lighthouse loops. Another person who had passed me earlier is huddled in the corner of the landing bent over. Lauren is leaning against the wall on the 24th floor landing. She laughs when she sees me. "I really should have trained for this. I always forget how hard it is. See you and Flip at the top."

30th floor. Three lighthouse loops. I speed up a little more, then at floor 32 it's time to pour it on. I push and pant, hear the cheers. I push harder, gasping, fighting for air, then burst up to floor 36, step on the timing pad, and emerge into lights and cheers. I bend down so a volunteer can place the medal on my neck, walk under the balloon arch and see Flip waving and grinning.

We high five. "Congratulations, hon. How did you do? How long were you waiting?"

Flip proudly shrugs. "Not long, maybe about five minutes. Is Mom far behind?"

"I passed her on the 24th floor. She said she needs to train more next year," I say, smiling.

Flip laughs. "She says that every year."

"She does, but she still shows up and climbs with us each year, such a good sport."

Flip and I wait a few more minutes, take a few selfies, then Lauren steps out of the stairwell, gets her medal, walks over to me and Flip. We all high five. I ask an older couple, "Would you please take a picture of me, my grandson, and daughter-in-law?"

The man takes my phone. "Of course!" As we hold up our medals and smile, the woman says, "You mean you climb together as a family?"

"We do! Lauren and I started five years ago, and Flip joined us a couple years later."

She smiles. "What a wonderful idea. You are so fortunate. Congratulations." She turns to her husband as they walk away. "Maybe we can try something like that next year."

The next day, Lauren texts me. "Results are posted. You placed 1st in your age group again and Flip placed 2nd in his. Congratulations!" I quickly check the results on my computer. Flip completed in 7:59, second place in the 10 to 18 male group. Lauren did fine at 16:16. My time was 12:14. I placed first but there were only two other women in the 70+ age group. And one was 81! Now that's inspiring.

One of my dreams is that someday there will be so many 70+ seniors that they will have to add an 80-89 age group rather than just lumping all the 70s-and-above into one group.

Turning 80 is still daunting. But then my 70s scared me when I was in my 60s. And look how things have turned out. More physical issues have popped up. I've slowed down, but I was never that fast in the first place. And winning has never been my goal. Just competing with myself and being understanding when I couldn't keep up with last year's time.

And the biggest surprise of all? My 70s have somehow become my *bonus decade*. So, what the heck. I'll stop fretting about my 80s, because who knows what's on the horizon? I'll just continue making every day count, never taking anything for granted, being grateful, taking risks, staying active, savoring moments, connecting with others, moving forward. Climbing high. Stepping up.

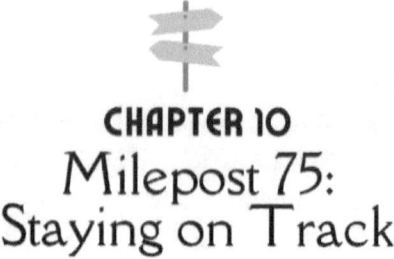

CHAPTER 10
Milepost 75:
Staying on Track

First event of my 75ᵗʰ year celebration: done! I sat on my Garmin ball at our kitchen table, eating breakfast, checking the list I had written out on a 4X6 card:

- February: The American Lung Association "Fight for Air Stair Climb" (736 steps, 36 stories)
- February: Melbourne Half Marathon
- February: St Augustine Lighthouse 5K
- March: Tomoka Park Half Marathon
- May: Sierra Club One Day Hike 50K
- May: Camino De Santiago 100K
- June through August: Open for training
- October: Grand Canyon one-day rim-to-rim hike
- October: Pink Army 5K
- October: Cottonmouth 5K
- November: Richmond Half Marathon
- December: Bulow Park Trail Run/Walk 13.6 miles
- December: Princess Place Preserve 5K

I had posted this list on my bulletin board, adjusting it as opportunities presented themselves. It served as a daily motivator to stay active and get out to walk just like I had hoped it would.

But even with all that motivation and inspiration I had started to drift away from earlier lessons I had learned. I was not being a good friend to my current or future self.

And later I would end up even sabotaging myself.

The following week we celebrated my 75th birthday. Jonathan and the boys came down for a low-key birthday weekend. We played rummy, walked, and cooked together. I chatted on the phone with Rachel, Rob, Jonathan, and Andrew. We feasted on our traditional birthday cake covered in Peanut M&M's and watched *Jeopardy!* together. Small and simple. My style. Our style.

The next event on my list was the half marathon down south in Melbourne, Florida with my friend Vicki from my WDW Marathon days.

From the very start, it was clear this would not be my best experience. There were wires and electrodes inserted across my lower back for my Inter-Stem implant pretest. My urologist told me it was okay for me to participate in this event as long as I kept all the electronic paraphernalia dry and intact. At first, I was good to go.

But around Mile 6, one wire had disengaged and was scratching my spine like a sharp needle pricking me with every step. I stopped, tried to stuff tissues on the irritation point, but nothing seemed to work. I just kept going, trying to ignore the pain as I soldiered on. Then it started to rain. I pulled out my poncho.

I struggled to embrace my usual event euphoria.

But, after a few more miles, the sun peaked out and I perked up. They served dill pickle juice at the 10 Mile Stop. Now that is something to celebrate! It's become one of my favorite energy boosts.

We had three more miles to finish this event on a high point. There was no pressure to walk fast since the full marathoners were on the same course. Vicki and I slowed way down and began reminiscing about our Disney Days and long history of happy walking memories. I even forgot about that scratching wire digging into my back.

On the final bridge, a woman ahead of us started yelling and pointing to the water. We looked down and saw three dolphins floating by, waving their fins at us. Now that was an unexpected delight!

Then at the end we had yet another surprise. The event organizers served strawberry shortcake right behind the finish line. What could be sweeter than that?

I had started this event slower than I would have liked and thought I had arrived at a good place by the end. But even with the final festivities I struggled to shake my frustration at our completion time of 4 hours and 30 minutes. Somehow, I was starting to lose some of my hard-earned perspective and determination to approach each event with joy and be satisfied with doing my best.

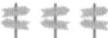

By the end of February, things had picked up. I had already checked three events off my list. Number four, the Tomoka Park Half Marathon, was coming up. I was excited. At first.

I usually enjoyed my training walks almost as much as participating in the actual event. But my joy had started fading and I found myself dragging during the final miles of each walk.

In the first week in March, I headed out fast and strong on another training walk. But on the way back, I stopped right in the middle of the trail. *Something just isn't right,* I realized. *I'm not enjoying this at all.* I started walking. Stopped again. *I love walking. I need to walk. Why do I feel so miserable?*

At first, I had shaken off the gloom as the sights and sounds of the trail embraced me. I basked in the vibrant hues of the flowers, enjoyed greeting other smiling walkers. But after walking eight miles, my smile and spirits had faded. My right IT Band was shrieking. My shoulders were hurting. No longer fun. Not in a good place. What was going on?

I sat down on a bench to think about how I got to this point.

Like just about everything else in my life, I was a late daily-walking starter. My passion for walking began in my mid-forties, but *daily* walking did not become part of my life until about 15 years later after my first hip-replacement surgery in my early sixties.

A key part of my rehab was to walk every day. First short walks, then a bit longer, always outside. My hip healed. I regained my strength. And discovered a new passion.

I soon realized that I didn't feel complete unless I could stride outside, see the sky, smell the air, feel the crunch of gravel, dirt, or snow under my feet, enveloped in nature with all my senses. A tree, a butterfly, a bush. Breeze, birds, insects.

After three more joint-replacement surgeries and yet another foot injury, I finally accepted that another Grand Canyon R2R2R was not in the cards. I modified my goal to a R2R. I ramped up my training walks for big events, especially half marathons and even shorter Grand Canyon hikes. But even when I was not training, I still walked every day with joy.

And when I walked longer distances training for a big event, the joy became even more intense, sometimes even palpable. The further I walked, the more I felt embraced by a mysterious bit of trail euphoria. Hard to describe—even understand.

But now I was feeling miserable on my longer training walks. I had lost that loving feeling.

I got up, walked another mile, stopped again, and didn't even pause my Apple Watch.

Then it dawned on me. Somewhere along the line I had started relying on my watch too much. Because it measured my pace, my walking *speed* had become an outsized goal. The end rather than a means to an end. I remembered how my focus on timing had even reduced my joy of the Melbourne Half Marathon.

That was it. I was walking for my watch, not for me.

I had to recapture my attitude of gratitude. To rediscover my joy of walking. That joy that pulled me out in nature every day.

A few days later, I was back on the trail training for Tomoka, walking longer distances at a *comfortable* speed, sometimes fast, sometimes slow, whatever felt good, continuing to build strength and endurance. I set distance goals but no longer let my pace numbers distract and interfere. I even stopped pushing *pause* when I stopped to chat with neighbors and pet their dear dogs. The IT-Band pain disappeared, along with my frustration. My shoulders relaxed. My joy returned.

Vicki drove up from Orlando to walk this half marathon with me. Her friend Jeanne joined us. We started at 6:30 in pitch dark through a cramped neighborhood street. The sun peaked out and we reached a smooth main road that took us up and over the Intracoastal Waterway bridge, in and out of the tantalizing tree-filled Tomoka Park. We chatted, sharing favorite travel stories. Jeanne was going to the Galapagos. I had hiked in Peru. We passed water stops and mile markers much faster than I anticipated. We continued through beautiful friendly neighborhoods along the water and back over ICW bridge to the finish line.

I felt good—and strong. When I finally looked at my watch, I saw I had walked 13.1 miles in 4 hours and 4 minutes with a pace of 18:38. My fastest half marathon pace since I had retired. Well, what do you know? What a pleasant surprise. I love competing against myself, so this was a huge win for me.

I also placed *first* in my age group, but that was *only* because there was no one else in the female 75 and older age group. Actually, I like having many women in this age group, both fast and slow, even if that means I come in at the end. It gives me hope for the future. More senior women, a louder voice, bigger presence, more inspiration, collegiality.

But I must admit, receiving that first-place plaque this year felt good. Especially since it now serves as a tangible reminder that when I walk in comfort and joy on my daily walks, I can usually walk with more ease in my occasional big events. And, big surprise, I may end up walking faster. But even if I don't, that's fine too.

Who knew? I found a new way to age adventurously by never losing the joy as I stay fit every day, every walk. I can track and measure as long as I remember to keep that information in perspective. I learned a new way to enjoy walking and staying active so I can be a *best friend forever* to my future self.

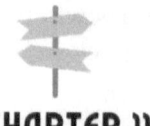

CHAPTER 11
Building Family Legacy
on One Day Hike

In 1954, Supreme Court Justice William O. Douglas and other passionate preservationists hiked along the *entire* 184.5-mile Chesapeake and Ohio Canal from Cumberland, Maryland to Washington, D.C. The National Park Service had wanted to turn this spectacular stretch of history into a highway. Justice Douglas and the others took this long walk to help prevent portions of the canal from being covered in pavement.

It worked! Their walk contributed to the establishment of the Chesapeake and Ohio National Historical Park in 1971. Douglas took one big step, inspired a community of followers, mounted a campaign, and made a difference.

Shortly after Rob and Rachel moved to Lexington Park for Rob's next US Navy assignment, Rachel discovered an event along this very same canal. And in 2011, she and Rob started their One Day Hike (ODH) journey.

That first year, they hiked most of the entire 100K, but couldn't complete the last five miles because Rob's feet were covered in blisters. The next year, they couldn't complete it because they both got sick.

Rachel had learned long ago that not finishing a hike did not mean giving it up. If they didn't make it the first time—or even the second or third time—they would learn, adjust, and try again. It's what we do. That's what they did. On their third attempt, they made it. 100K. 62.2 miles. One day.

Sponsored by the Sierra Club, the One Day Hike began in 1974. At first it was 100K. Some years later, the 50K (31.1 miles) was added, with both hikes merging and ending at Harpers Ferry, another national historical park. About 30 miles of the hike is along the C&O Canal towpath.

At the beginning of 2014, during my first full year of retirement and the year I turned 70, I said to Rachel. "This is such a neat hike. I would love to do the 50K. What do you think?" (I later learned that 2014 was the 60th anniversary of Justice Douglas' hike. How fortuitous.).

"Great idea!" Rachel said. "Jonathan said he might be interested in hiking the 50K now that he's old enough. The two of you could do it together. Maybe Dad and Andrew can meet us at the end in Harpers Ferry. Dad will love alone time with Andrew. And you will love this hike!"

What a perfect opportunity to build a new hiking legacy on the ODH to balance our experiences at the Grand Canyon! Mike Darzi, the co-chair and volunteer coordinator of the ODH, sent out engaging emails that made remote training easy and fun. We couldn't train with the folks who lived in the DC area, but we could use Mike's emails as our virtual training guide, building our strength and endurance as the weekly hikes became progressively longer.

In April 2014 it all came together. As planned, Rachel and Rob started the 100K in Georgetown. Arnie drove Jonathan and me to White's Ferry to start the 50K. He and Andrew drove to Harpers Ferry to spend a memorable grandpa-grandson day together, exploring, chatting, and buying food for the very hungry hikers.

The ODHs between 2014 and 2018 added a brand-new dimension to our lives.

At mid-morning, April 2014, Jonathan and I stood in the White's Ferry starting area adjusting our bibs. He was the youngest hiker at 13. I was 70, not the oldest but close. We chatted with a trio of three old men (close to my age). One of them offered wisdom and encouragement. "Grandma and grandson—what a great team. You should be fine. We're getting slower, but we keep hiking it every year and we love it every time. Make sure you stop and eat at each of the rest stops, drink enough water, and be sure to have fun. We'll probably see you at the end."

We were nervous until we hit the trail. Jonathan noticed a group of six turtles congregated along a log in the canal, sunning themselves. We talked a little. Walked in silence for a few miles. Talked some more. Soon we arrived at Monocacy at 10.9 miles, the first support station.

We checked in and out with the smiling, helping volunteers and got back on the trail. Sometimes Jonathan would point something out. Sometimes I would. Most of the time he listened to his iPod. I listened to the birds, the wind in the trees, my own thoughts. We were comfortable in our own space.

After we had checked in and moved on from Point of Rocks at 17.1 miles, I noticed Jonathan was limping. "Are you okay?"

"I'm starting to chafe, and my foot is hurting too," he admitted. "I think it's my arches."

"I have some toilet paper," I told him. "Let me roll some sheets together and make little arch pads for your shoes to see if that helps."

"Okay," he agreed. We stopped and he tucked the little TP pillows under each arch.

Jonathan is our oldest grandson. He taught me and Arnie a great deal about dealing with him on his terms. He helped us become better and more respectful grandparents, meeting him where he was at. I was aware of my boundaries in terms of offering some help and support. I could help with his feet, but I knew better than to discuss his personal, private problem with chafing. He walked gingerly, still struggling. I fervently hoped somebody at the next rest station could help him.

We moved slowly, trying to focus on enjoying the sights and

sounds. He did his best to cope. I did my best to keep things normal. "Jonathan, listen, we can hear car noise on the road and trains on the tracks. We can hear our feet clomping on the trail and water flowing in the Potomac River. What a nice confluence of moving sounds."

"That's cool," Jonathan agreed. "It's a nice distraction."

I looked ahead, saw balloons bouncing and people coming together. "There's Brunswick! We've hiked 23.7 miles! Let's check in with the medical volunteers. I'm sure they can help you."

Caring and capable volunteers immediately took charge. They accessed their first aid tools to treat and reduce the pain of his blisters and cushion his arches. One of the men took him over by a porta potty and gave him some paper towels and powder to help ease the painful chafing in his crotch.

They saw the determination and pain etched in his young, beautiful face. They pushed through his boundaries and did everything they could to help him feel better, body and soul.

"I know from many years of volunteering at this stop that the best thing to perk you up is a bag of cookies," said one smiling, sweet woman who walked over to where we were sitting on the bench in the first aid area. "Eat a few now and take the rest with you."

Jonathan managed to give her a big smile. I nodded. "Thank you." These ODH guardian angels nourished us, made us stronger.

As we sat, I thought back to that first Grand Canyon 50/24 when Rachel and I sat facing each other on the picnic bench at Phantom Ranch after she had received nourishment from a total stranger—our first guardian angel. It was decision time. "Do we stop and rest, maybe wait until morning?" I asked. "Or do we push on and hike up the South Rim? It's your choice." That was Rachel's Grand Canyon moment.

Now, almost 25 years later, as Jonathan and I sat on a bench, nourished and feeling a bit stronger, I asked: "Do we stop here and get a ride to the end? Or do we hike? It's your choice."

"I'm okay. I'm going to finish this on my own two feet," he said. The same choice his mom had made those many years ago. Would this become his One Day Hike moment?

We rested for a while longer in the care and comfort of Brunswick. A few more hikers walked by. "Jonathan, look at all the 100K bibs. I bet your mom and dad will catch up with us on this final portion."

"Great. We can go now. I'm ready." We checked out of Brunswick and got back on the trail with 7.4 miles to go. The sun set an hour later. We turned on our flashlights and quietly celebrated each mile marker.

Jonathan started walking slower, kept turning and looking back. He wanted his parents. We were both getting tired. A few other hikers passed us on the trail. "Are you okay?" they asked.

"We're fine, thanks for checking," I responded. "Have a good hike."

We heard people talking behind us. Saw flashlights bouncing up the path. "I think that's Mom and Dad," said Jonathan.

He was right. Rachel and Rob caught up to us. "We checked to see what time you left Brunswick. I'm so glad we caught up with you!" Rachel exclaimed. Then she looked at Jonathan. "Is everything okay?"

"Well, my feet are pretty sore and I'm chafing really bad," Jonathan said. Rob took him over to the side of the trail and they talked quietly. Rob took Jonathan's backpack and they hiked on ahead. Jonathan perked up as soon as his dad was hiking beside him, and his mom nearby.

Rachel and I hiked behind them, quietly sharing our stories. It felt good to be together as we hiked the final four miles. Each of us was in varying degrees of pain and exhaustion, but we knew with every step we were getting closer to the end.

Finally, we climbed the spiral staircase, walked across the bridge, trudged up the hill, and stepped into the bright lights and cheers of Bolivar Community Center!

We checked in and did our best to smile at Mike Darzi as he took our finisher photos. We told him about the caring and helpful volunteers at every rest stop, especially Brunswick. And then, as if on cue, one volunteer handed us our treasured finisher patches and another team of volunteers served us pizza and chili!

Our aching muscles and swollen feet started demanding attention just as Arnie and Andrew picked us up and drove to a nearby hotel. It was hard to sleep that night. It would take a while for our bodies to heal, but not our spirits.

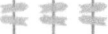

The next morning, we ate a gigantic breakfast at the local IHOP. I'm not sure Jonathan recognized it at the time, but the rest of us knew this would be more than just a memory for him. It would be a touch point, a reference, his very own moment. When he was only 13, the youngest on the trail, and in lots of pain, he refused to give up. He discovered his deep well of strength and determination that would arm him with the knowledge that he could succeed at anything he put his mind to. Years later in Army Basic Training, he was faced with a big challenge, and he persevered. He knew he had the capacity to succeed. That he would not give up, not ever.

This hike would be a touchstone in Jonathan's life just like Rachel's Grand Canyon experience was in hers. Both involved big steps that made a lifelong difference. I had been given the gift of sharing a life-altering, strength-building event with my daughter and now with my firstborn grandson. From generation to generation.

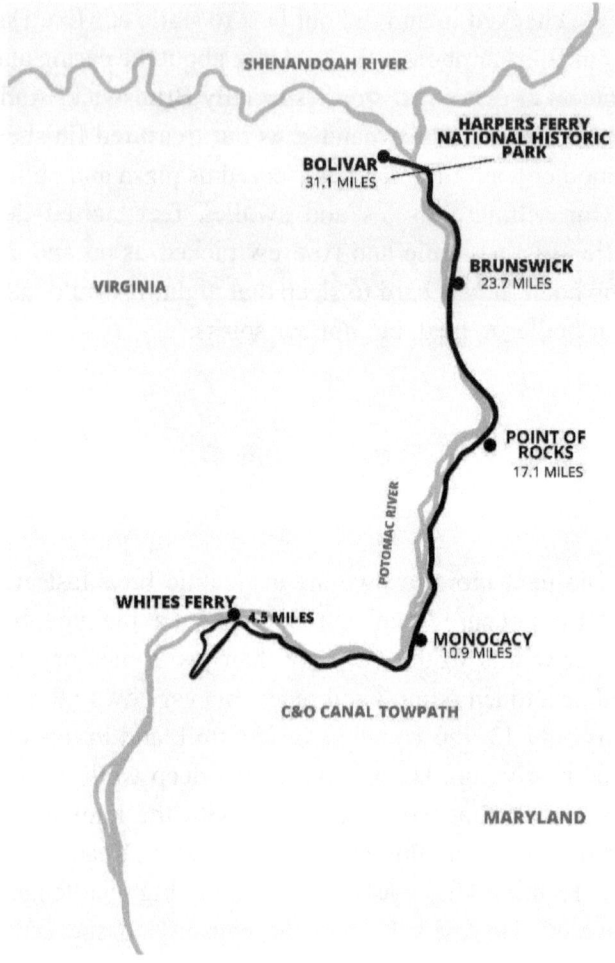

We skipped 2015 because Arnie and I were in the middle of moving to Florida, then hit the trail again in 2016. I had broken my foot earlier that year in March, but it was healing well and I felt confident I could complete the ODH if I walked just a bit slower. Arnie decided to stay home in Florida, Andrew was old enough to participate, and Rachel and Rob decided to hike the 50K so we could be together, start and finish.

At White's Ferry, I asked the kids to hike ahead since it would be easier and more comfortable for me to walk my own pace with no pressure to keep up. They could eat and relax while they waited for me in the cheery collegial comfort of Bolivar Community Center.

My training hikes had gone well, but when my broken foot started to hurt around 10 miles, I decided to play it safe and end my hike at Monocacy. The ODH was just three months before our Inca Trail Trek. I did not want to risk breaking it again.

I waited at Monocacy until I caught a ride with Rob Anderson, the volunteer transportation director who was getting ready to drive to the Brunswick rest stop and on to the Bolivar finish. He and his wife had hiked the Inca Trail a few years earlier, so we had lots to talk about during the drive. I peppered him with questions. He happily shared stories and tips. "You and your daughter will be fine. I've seen you both on the trail." We started that brief car ride as strangers. By the end, Rob and I formed a bond that has grown stronger with each passing year.

While we were in the car, Rachel texted: Andrew injured his ankle just after Point of Rocks. We're still hiking but we will have to stop at Brunswick. Rob and Jonathan are fine, have gone ahead.

I asked *my new friend* Rob to drop me off at Brunswick. Soon *son-in-law* Rob and Jonathan came hiking down the trail. Later, we saw Rachel and Andrew. He was barely able to walk. Rob and Jonathan headed out to hike the final 7.4 miles. Rachel, Andrew, and I caught a ride with another volunteer and got to Bolivar Community Center in time to cheer Rob and Jonathan as they walked through the door shortly after 9:00. Each of us became more attached and attracted to ODH magic. And we learned that as long as we started and celebrated at the end together, we could create shared memories.

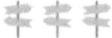

We all knew we'd be back on the trail the following year, 2017. And we were. The kids headed out ahead of me as we had planned. I had fun hiking at my own pace, being alone with my thoughts, enjoying each sight and sound. Walking, watching, wondering, I passed the hours in my private, peaceful meditation.

When I left Brunswick after being given several tasty, salty, and sweet treats by those amazing volunteers, I figured I could easily complete the final 7.4 miles and finish by 11:00 p.m. But after hiking three more miles, I hit a wall. *I'm less than five miles from the end and I can barely move. What's going on? I must not have eaten enough*, I thought as I grabbed some snacks from my backpack. At this point, it was tough to swallow, but I shoved a few bites of a granola bar into my mouth and pushed forward a couple more miles.

A bike patrol volunteer rode up. "Are you okay? Mike radioed me from Bolivar. Your daughter is worried."

I smiled. "Thank you for checking. I'm fine, just tired. Please ask Mike to let Rachel know I'm okay."

"Here, eat this banana and drink another bottle of water. Are you sure you're okay? You have less than two miles left."

"I am. I will make it. This snack is just what I need. Thank you." I kept going, feeling better. Just a little worried I might not make the end time of midnight, even though I had comfortably beat the cut-off times at each of the support stations. I needed to get to the bridge. I needed to walk up that final hill.

I kept walking, straining to see that magical mile marker just before the spiral staircase. Then I saw a flashlight heading my way. It was Rob! "Sandi, you're almost at the bridge. Give me your backpack. Let me help you. We were impressed with your pace when you checked out of Brunswick. But when it was an hour after we figured you'd finish, Rachel got worried. The bike patrol volunteer radioed Mike you were on your way and were still smiling. What happened?"

"I was fine and then just bonked. I'm sure I didn't eat enough. So sorry you had to come back down the hill, but I'm glad to see you. How did everyone else do?"

"Everyone is fine. Let's get across the bridge and I can help you finish."

We crossed the bridge and started up the hill. I put my hand on Rob's shoulder, happy for his support and soft chatter. "All those training hikes we started doing in January paid off. The boys were amazing. We may need to get some orthotics for Andrew to help deal with his ankle issues, but he did great even with his foot pain. How are you feeling?"

"I'm fine, Rob, just tired and a little sore. Thanks so much for coming to help me."

"Well, look at it this way, I'm helping both you and Rachel." Just then we looked up and saw the lights of the Bolivar Community Center at the top of the hill.

Someone was walking down toward us. "Hi, Grandma. Are you okay? Can I help too?"

"Oh yes, Jonathan. If you walk on my other side so I can put my hand on your shoulder, that would be great. Thank you."

It was one of those times when something is so overwhelming, I can't absorb the power of the moment in real time. My world slowed almost to a stop. I could feel Jonathan's strength traveling up my left arm and Rob's steady support traveling up my right. My chest tightened. I blinked away tears burning my eyes.

Then real time returned. We stepped up to the door. Jonathan and Rob stood back so I could walk in alone. As soon as I signed in and received my finisher's patch, we gathered for a family photo.

Later I was able to mix my disappointment with perspective. I wasn't at my best, but still, I *had* hiked on that incredible trail for more than 14 hours straight, starting at White's Ferry at 10:00 a.m. and walking into Bolivar at 12:15 am. I had spent all those hours in a spiritual place, surrounded by nature, encouraged and supported by volunteers, family, even other hikers. My heart was full.

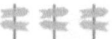

When I go into the claustrophobic tube of a CT scan, all I do is think back to this hike. To the hours and miles of walking alone in peace and beauty. My heart rate slows, I relax and bask in the peaceful memories of my long walk in the woods.

In 2018, Rachel, Rob, and the boys hiked almost every weekend in Maryland. I trained hard with daily walks of 2-3 miles and at least 20 weekend training hikes of 6 to 18 miles in Florida. We all completed it in 2017. No injuries. A few blisters. A ton of memories. This hike had become more than an annual event. More than a long hike. It had become a lifestyle. We train, we plan, pack, and travel. We hike. We savor, celebrate, learn, and adjust.

In April, I flew to Maryland for my two-week spring visit with the kids. Then we drove to Rockville to spend the night before starting the hike the next morning. We checked in at the hotel and headed out to the grocery store to pick up a few last-minute snacks. As we walked around the aisles, I felt weak. *This is crazy. I have been feeling so good and strong. What is happening to me?* I said to myself as I tried to ignore it, suspecting it may be a urinary tract infection, even though I had never had one before. I tried to shake it off again, telling myself I'd feel better in the morning after a good night's sleep. I didn't.

My mind was racing, trying to figure out how this could have happened. It finally dawned on me that the possibility of UTI was one of the potential side effects of my Botox treatment for urinary urge incontinence. I solved the mystery, but by morning I knew hiking the ODH would not be in the cards for me this year.

"Oh, Mom, I'm so sorry! You have trained so hard. Are you sure you don't want to try it?" Rachel asked.

"No, hon. I know my body. This hike is challenging enough for me when I feel great. I hate to stay behind, especially when I trained so hard and felt so ready. But this is the right and reasonable thing to do. Please have fun and text a few updates and pictures so I can be with you in spirit. Don't worry. I'll be fine."

Rachel, Rob, and the boys rode the shuttle to White's Ferry. I slept for a while, then texted Uber to go to Urgent Care and the pharmacy. I went back to the hotel, took my first dose of antibiotics, and went back to bed. I woke up a few hours later, feeling rested and even a bit stronger.

I can't hike the 50K, but I'm certainly strong enough to salvage the remains of this day, I said to myself. I checked the driving distance to Bolivar Community Center at Harpers Ferry. *It's just 45 minutes from here. The price is reasonable. I can Uber and meet the kids at the end, celebrate, and shuttle back to the hotel with them. I don't have to miss the entire experience!*

I thought about my UTI. The Botox injection had worked, but it worked too well, so I had trouble fully emptying my bladder. But I didn't dwell. Instead, I settled into gratitude. *It's a good time to be aging. We have so many medical options to deal with issues like this that women in Mom's generation just had to live with.*

I arrived at Bolivar in late afternoon and checked in with Mike to see if he needed any extra volunteer help at the finish line. "We have enough help here, but later on it would be great if you can help the volunteers on the hill cheer and guide the hikers as they drag themselves up that last vertical mile."

It dawned on me that I could hike down our dreaded final hill and see everything I missed when we trudge up this last portion in total darkness. As I hiked down the hill in daylight, I realized there was so much more to that hill than what had been squeezed into the narrow beam of my flashlight. Now I could see historic buildings, a beautiful old church, fascinating window decorations, monuments, Harpers Ferry markers. I walked down to the Potomac Bridge surrounded by delightful sights. What fun!

When I saw more hikers crossing the bridge and climbing the hill, I walked back up and introduced myself to a young woman standing a few blocks down from Bolivar. She was delighted to have some company. We spent the next two hours chatting with each other and cheering the hikers as they passed. "Congratulations! Just a few more blocks. Someone will show you to where you turn left. You'll see the lights of Bolivar in just a few minutes. Congratulations! Good job!"

I made the best of this day. I could cry or cheer. Maybe the tears would come later, but for now I would celebrate the accomplishment of others and share their joy.

Darkness descended as I headed back to the Community Center to wait for the kids. About an hour later they walked through the door. A joyful ending as I greeted Rachel, Rob, Jonathan, and Andrew and listened to their hiking stories.

Andrew's ankle issues had been resolved. Now he was leading, not lagging. He had started creating his own legacy on the ODH. And many years later he would even more fully embrace hiking and walking family adventures, leading the way again.

I learned a valuable lesson about discovering fragments of delight that can easily get hidden in the detritus of disappointment. Even though my day did not go as planned, I was able to find new reasons to celebrate.

I was getting pretty good at this!

What I didn't know was that next year I would end up writing a new ODH chapter to our hiking story that would provide even more lessons.

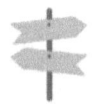

CHAPTER 12
Fewer Miles and More Lessons on the 50K One Day Hike

It was 2019. Hiking the ODH, a major item on my 75th year celebration list, was falling into place.

Until it wasn't.

But as this journey unfolded, I learned to embrace two life-changing paradigms that would help guide me as I continued moving forward, aging and staying active.

I learned that *just* is a welcome and necessary four-letter word.

I also learned that while *all the way* is a compelling goal, sometimes *less is more* and *Plan B* can be viable options.

Another dream had emerged way back in 2010 when I saw *The Way*, the movie staring Martin Sheen about hiking the entire 500 miles of the Camino de Santiago. I wanted to do this! But, since I had viewed this hike as an *all or nothing* adventure, I acknowledged reality and let that dream recede. Not feasible or reasonable for me.

Then, back in the summer of 2018, I read *Two Steps Forward*, another story about hiking the entire Camino de Santiago. It renewed my interest in that trail. I loved the book and passed it on to Cathy, my new Florida book club buddy. She read it and came up with a totally *novel* idea. "We could do just a portion of this hike! My friend Jane would love to do it too. Can you find another hiker so we could make it a foursome? Jane and I think we would need at least a year or more to train, so maybe we shoot for 2020. What do you think?"

I laughed at myself for never even considering hiking just a section of the Camino. Then I called Nancy Brown, the leader of our temple book club in Columbus. We had walked a half marathon together in Ohio. And a few years later we even met in Arizona to participate in "The Bisbee 1,000 Great Stair Climb" near Tucson. We both planned to be in that area visiting family and friends. We were both intrigued with this unique 4.5-mile event in an old mining town built on the side of a mountain. The entire town of Bisbee is connected by flights of steps leading from one level to another. Some clever folks had decided to create an event based on the town's unique design. Climbing 1000 steps up nine staircases connected by winding roads throughout historic Bisbee just sounded too cool to miss—like traveling to a different country!

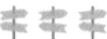

There's that saying: "Fences make good neighbors." My life mantra had become something different: "Walking makes good friends." I called Nancy and asked if she would be interested in this new adventure. She was in. I had a Camino Comrade! As a 76-year-old woman who walks at least 15 miles every week, Nancy was the perfect fourth member of our *Old Lady Camino Hiking Team*. Our ages ranged from 67 to 76. We all walked. We all loved to travel. What could go wrong?

The summer passed. A few days after I returned from Israel, Cathy sent an email telling me that she and Jane had just heard a presentation from a lady who had hiked part of the Camino using a walker. They were so inspired, they immediately considered moving our trip from 2020 to 2019. "I know I'm popping this on you right after you got home, but what do you think?"

I had to decide quickly so we could start planning. The ideal time would be early May to avoid the summer heat and crowds.

But I still didn't know the date of the 2019 One Day Hike.

Time passed. Pressure mounted. Cathy sent another email saying that we could fly to Madrid on May 7, spend a few days acclimating and seeing the sights, take the train to Sarria, and start the hike May 11.

I checked with Nancy. The dates worked for her. I had to decide quickly so I took the plunge and agreed to go for it. Jane contacted Macs Adventure and secured our spots. We paid our deposits and received our confirming email.

We were all set. Until the next day. That's when Mike Darzi sent out an email explaining that due to unforeseen scheduling issues, the date of the hike had been moved back to May 4.

May 4?! This would mean I'd be hiking the 50K just a few days before traveling to Spain. Yikes. I had planted these seeds of disruption when I gave Cathy the book. Now I had to reap what I had sowed. Obviously the easiest and most rational thing would be to just skip the hike for next year and replace it with the Camino trek. But I could not do that. Next year might be my last chance to hike the ODH.

I rattled off the situation to Arnie. "This will be tight. Are you okay if I leave from Rachel's right after the ODH rather than flying home first? That means I'll be gone for almost four weeks."

My dear husband listened carefully and responded calmly, helping me settle down. "I know how much you want to do this. The weather is nice here and Jonathan has already made plans to come down and spend a few weekends here with the boys. Are you sure you'll be okay with such a short break between hikes?"

"I think so. Since we will have two days in Madrid and a few travel days, I would not start hiking the Camino until the following Saturday. I should be rested and recovered from the 50K by then." Arnie smiled. He did not disagree, trusting me to eventually figure out how unrealistic that was.

By January of 2019 I had already completed 10 training hikes ranging from 6 to 10 miles, along with walking 2-4 miles every day. My feet were doing fine, especially since I had received my injection of Prolia, that shot that gave me a huge infusion of bone strength and confidence. But just to be sure, I still said a little "foot mantra" every time I went out for a walk. "Be strong; go the distance; don't break."

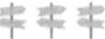

I walked, listening to my *step, step, step,* knowing my feet were getting stronger with every hike. But then those encouraging steps started sounding more like *stop, stop, stop.* My feet were trying to tell me something. I refused to listen. It didn't make sense. I was following the plan, gradually building my foot strength by steadily increasing miles. This is what I needed to do to be able to comfortably hike 10-12 miles for 6 days straight on the Camino after hiking the ODH. I couldn't possibly stop. I had come too far. The *stop, stop, stop* grew louder. It finally became too hard to ignore.

I stopped. Reality set in. This was not about my feet. It was about my body. I was trying to do too much in too little time. *It's crazy to think I could hike 31.1 miles and then start my next trip just two days later. I know how much this hike takes out of me and how long it takes me to recover.* But my heart still responded, *I don't want to miss the ODH again! I want the joy of hiking this trail, the volunteers, other hikers, all the sights and sounds. I'm trained. I'm ready. I have worked so hard for this. I do not want to stop and skip the ODH! I want it all!*

Then, other forces emerged that were beyond my control. One of the bridges on the C&O Canal toll path had washed out just before Brunswick. Mike and his team adjusted this year's route and established the endpoint at Point of Rocks with a loopback to Monocacy to add the miles and avoid the broken bridge.

So, we'd just repeat one section. No interesting hike to Brunswick. No hike through the dark forest. No walk across the Potomac Bridge at Harpers Ferry. No dragging ourselves up the long hill to the Bolivar Community Center.

It's not just the number of miles that makes this hike so meaningful. It's the whole journey.

I was bummed.

Rachel wasn't.

"Mom," she said, "this route change is perfect! You can hike to Point of Rocks—the new end point—and just stay there waiting for us to do the entire thing. That way you can have all the trail experiences that are available this year. We will do the loopback while you rest and wait for us, and we can celebrate together just like we did last year."

Well, what do you know! I could be reasonable, cut out some miles, and still spend precious time on the ODH. The route was adjusted for this year, so I could certainly adjust my approach and avoid overdoing it right before leaving for Spain.

The following month Rachel, Rob, Jonathan, and Andrew headed off from White's Ferry at their fast pace and I took my time to walk with no pressure since I was doing my own abbreviated ODH. On earlier hikes I would just sit for a few minutes on the short wall of a lock by the trail shortly before Monocacy. But this time I walked down to the section between the 8-foot walls of the lock. I stood close, placed my hands flat on the stones, appreciating the artistic beauty of these mighty walls crafted by skilled stone masons in the early 1800s. Memories of warm rocks at Machu Picchu and the Western Wall filled my head.

As I rested my hands and savored the heat, a bit of history popped into my head. The original intent of the C&O Canal was that it would provide a transportation system from the Ohio River in Pittsburgh all the way to D.C.

But here's the deal. Although the Chesapeake and Ohio Canal provided a vital coal pipeline from the Allegheny Mountains to Washington D.C., it never achieved its *original* intent of starting at Pittsburgh. Never went the distance. And today, neither would I. The Canal and I had something in common. Nice! I would have never had this moment if I had been fixated on completing the entire 31.1 miles this year.

After walking another mile or so I treated myself to another side trip at the mammoth Monocacy Aqueduct. I knew I'd have time to stop and get a good look at this historic structure, so I had done a little more homework. This "water bridge" that carried canal boats over rivers and streams was one of eleven aqueducts on the C&O Canal. I strolled down to the river to get a closer look at the seven symmetrical arches constructed with artful precision. It was designed by chief engineer Benjamin Wright who was also the lead engineer of the Erie Canal. And Monocacy is considered one of the most beautiful and the largest of the canal aqueducts.

I had hiked over this magnificent monument many times, but this was the first year I did more than just glance and move quickly on. I sat for a while longer watching the waterway moving slowly, gently under its arches. Appreciating the pause. Feeling the flow.

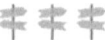

I stepped back on the trail and soon saw the kids walking toward me as they headed on their loopback. We stopped. I gave them a few snacks and dampened paper towels. Rachel sprayed me with bug spray. We cheered each other. They headed down to their second stop at Monocacy and I hiked on to Point of Rocks.

As I walked, I thought about how the ODH had become a facet of our lives—a legacy, a part of our history. The kids would have many years of going the distance. I didn't know how many I had left. But I did know I would show up as long as I could. As a hiker. As a volunteer, or simply to cheer and support my family.

I reached Point of Rocks, my personal endpoint, tired but delighted with my 19.5-mile hike that included sweet side trips off the beaten path. Best of all I had one more year to be with my family at the beginning, end, and even the middle of the One Day Hike.

I learned that complications can easily turn into opportunities to be creative, even learn. While completing the entire event or journey is a great goal, sometimes completing just a portion is wiser, even worthier. My Grand Canyon lessons and experiences returned and resonated. My active life had started with a DNF when Rachel and I turned around on the North Rim trail. There is a time to turn back or trim back and a time to push on.

If something happens that prevents me from finishing a full event even after months of training, that training is never wasted. Every one of those training walks was good for me, my body and soul.

I also learned to fully embrace "just" as a word that *describes* my accomplishment but does not *diminish* it. This insight is gaining traction as I get older. I still say, I *just* walk (not run); I do *just* a half marathon (not a full marathon). And this works, as long as I add, "It's good enough for me. It's good as gold."

And so this year I hiked *just* 19.5 miles of the ODH (not the full 31.1 miles). And in those 19.5 miles, I discovered the joy of my first "Plan B" adventure.

CHAPTER 13
Walking in Madrid

"Oh my gosh, we missed the Bosch!" Jane said just as we started to leave the Prado, the iconic Spanish national art museum in Madrid. This cavernous and majestic hall of artistic delights was on our list of must-see sights.

Jane, Cathy, and I were exhausted from our red-eye flight from JFK to Madrid. We had already spent two hours checking out our favorite paintings and sculptures, but Jane was adamant. We had to turn back and see one more. Once we stepped into the small, almost vacant gallery, we saw what Jane's fuss was about. Hieronymus Bosch's *Garden of Earthly Delights*, a mammoth 7 X 13-foot triptych, dominated the room and was filled with tiny, intricate scenes, almost too much to absorb.

The left section depicted the creation story with a creator draped in a flowing robe, a naked man and woman, blue sky, green grass, even the notorious tree. Some familiar animals roamed through the grass, but most creatures were other-worldly. Buildings and mountains defied description. The right section was dark, tortured, dismal, populated with people and disconcerting objects. The middle and most captivating section was filled with dozens of people, creatures, architectural wonders, surreal and magical. Jane was right. We could not miss this.

When we finally left the Prado, Cathy turned to me. "We can see Picasso's *Guernica* in the Sofia Reina tomorrow. I know that was a big thing on your list."

Jane agreed. "Contemporary art is not my favorite, but I'm

sure we will enjoy touring that museum too."

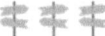

In some ways Cathy and Jane are like an old married couple. And, since Nancy could not join us due to family illness, I was the third wheel. They were a pair, a team. It would be like asking twins to suddenly become triplets. This trip would be different for all of us.

We will make this work, I reassured myself. *It will be a collegial adventure within the Camino adventure and an opportunity to build a new relationship with two women I've never traveled with before. We love to walk, hike, and travel. We can strengthen that bond during this trip.*

Building relationships with other active women has become even more important to me as I've traveled through my 70s. At this age, it's not that easy to find other women who enjoy exploring new geographical and physical domains. It's even more challenging to create new relationships.

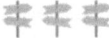

At this point, I was pretty set in my ways. I suspected Cathy and Jane were too. Now we had an opportunity to exercise our accommodation muscles as we explored this new territory together.

I was the oldest at 75 and stood a full head and shoulders above both women. Jane was 67, brown hair pulled back in a pony tail, an experienced traveler, sturdy, a force of nature. Cathy was 68, petite and strong. She wore her dark brown hair short with heavy bangs that framed her smiling round face. She had liver transplant surgery 19 years earlier and even more fully embraced life ever since. Cathy was full of grace and gratitude. Once when

I commented on my slower pace as we walked together, she replied, "I am slower these days as well, but what matters is that we are vertical and moving!"

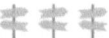

The next day was our bonus day. We walked across the street to the Sofia Reina. While it had worked for us to stay together at the Prado, it made more sense to split up here. Cathy and Jane wanted to explore every room while I preferred to linger in just a few. We agreed to meet up in the sculpture garden in two and a half hours.

I headed straight to my reunion with Picasso's *Guernica*. As I walked through the vaulted hallways, my thoughts traveled back to when Arnie and I lived in Queens, New York, the first year we were married, 1969. We felt like strangers in a strange land, so different from Arizona. The weather, the culture, the pace. Even the fast, boisterous way of speaking was quite different from our more laid-back manner in Arizona. The corner breakfast café had a shouting server behind the counter. Shoppers fought over grocery carts at our neighborhood supermarket. And outside our window, we could hear drivers honking their horns all hours of the day. It was loud, busy, fascinating.

Almost every weekend, we hopped on the subway to Manhattan. One day in the Museum of Modern Art, Arnie had walked ahead of me into another gallery and came rushing back. "Sandi, come here. You have got to see this." I walked around the corner with him, saw the majestic and moving anti-war painting and stood glued in awe. Through our many years of marriage I will always remember how it felt to stand close to Arnie and gaze at *Guernica* in MOMA in NYC.

Now I was in Madrid, walking toward the gallery where *Guernica* had returned home. My heart started racing as I stepped into a corridor filled with preliminary studies and sketches of each portion of the painting. Finally, I walked through the door and there it was!

The painting looked *exactly* as I remembered it—except for one thing. Somehow my mind had created a memory of this same painting in vivid color. But there it was, in black, grey, and white.

Since I had not planned to walk through this entire museum, I gave myself the gift of time to pause and reflect. Maybe I remembered *Guernica* in color because I wanted to.

As I sat and pondered this conundrum a bit more, I remembered that Arnie and I had some tough times in New York adjusting to each other, to married life, to life away from family and friends. But now, almost all my memories of that year are of the good things. I guess as I grow older, I tend to color most parts of my past with beautiful hues. Even the hard times have soft technicolor linings.

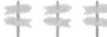

After roaming the museum, I sat on a bench in the sculpture garden, watching the breeze gently move the eight blades of an Alexander Calder mobile. *I just spent the last two hours wandering through beauty, traveling back in time, meeting up with a sweet artifact from my past, and this day has just begun.*

I stood up to go meet Cathy and Jane so we could finish making the most of our bonus day in Madrid before taking the train to Sarria tomorrow.

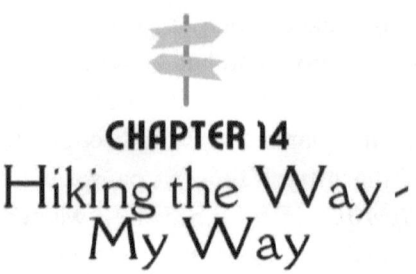

CHAPTER 14
Hiking the Way - My Way

Day One

I woke at 6:00 a.m. I did my usual ten minutes of Tai Chi and yoga exercises, set up my hiking poles, repacked my bag, and joined Cathy and Jane for breakfast at 7:00. Macs Adventure, our touring company, had made all our hotel reservations. Breakfast was included in our package. We were responsible for lunch and dinner.

I had been concerned I might not get enough protein at breakfast and had even packed a jar of crunchy peanut butter. The dining room was filled with trays of yogurt, pastries, hard-boiled eggs, oatmeal, more pastries all artfully displayed. One cake was even decorated with a powdered-sugar stencil of the Celtic Cross.

I broke from my usual black coffee habit and drank two small cups of *café con leche,* getting even more protein with the additional milk.

Jane, who had taken the lead in organizing and planning our trip, had ordered scallop shells for us, explaining, "It's a tradition for pilgrims to wear these shells on their backpacks."

She had also sent us the requirements for the official *Compostela* certificate we could obtain in Santiago. The two requirements that stuck with me were that we would have to walk at least the final 100KM on the trail and get at least two *cellos* (stamps) in our Camino Passport every day. We could get our passports stamped at each place we stayed and at each café, plus shops, churches, and roadside stands.

I returned to my room, freshened up, tied my scallop shell on my backpack, and left the unopened jar of peanut butter on the dresser. We dropped off our luggage in the lobby. The desk clerk carefully stamped and dated each of our passports with the date of 11/05/19. "Wait a minute! It's not November and it's not the 5th." Then it dawned on me. In Spain, the standard format is day first, then month. Just another delightful nuance of traveling and learning.

"Look!" said Cathy. "I wonder if all the stamps will be different." This *cello* was a black outline of a traditional pilgrim with a broad hat, staff, and a scallop shell around his neck with SARRIA printed across the bottom.

We left the hotel at 8:00 am and headed to Rua Major which would lead us to the main trail. We strolled alone and along this cobblestone road bordered by multi-colored buildings.

Jane turned left into a courtyard and discovered a statue of King Afonso IX of Leon and Galicia sitting on a throne, looking stern, wearing a tall crown, clutching a giant sword. She asked Cathy to pose by the statue, holding her hiking pole as a scepter in her right hand, looking quite regal herself. Facebook picture perfect.

We climbed down a long flight of steps and stepped onto the main trail. At 8:30 we saw our first *official* km marker, a 4-foot-high tapered block monument. Its flat top served as a receptacle for rocks and other small treasures placed as offerings by those who passed by. Almost every other monument would be the same. On the front was a royal blue tile etched with a yellow scallop shell laying on its side, rays pointing forward. Under the tile, a yellow arrow pointed in the same direction. A small metal rectangular plate under the arrow was inscribed with tiny km numbers out to three decimal points. We translated the kms to miles, dividing by 1.6.

As we stood and gazed at our first yellow arrow, we were

confident we would not get lost. Ivan told us so.

Yesterday when we checked into Hotel Alfonso, Jane asked Ivan, the desk clerk, "How easy is it to get lost?" Ivan smiled big. "It is not *impossible* but *very difficult* to get lost. You will see the yellow arrows and you will follow them." He looked at Jane who still had a slight wrinkle in her brow. She was not convinced. So Ivan continued, "You will see yellow arrows as soon as you hit the main trail, and you also have your guidebook. Follow the arrows. You will not get lost," he said, looking straight at Jane. Her brow unfurled, her face relaxed and settled into the hint of a grin. Ivan took a big breath and nodded his head, satisfied he had fully completed his task of properly checking us in and calming us down.

Back on the trail, we stopped just a few minutes later to check out a sculpture.

It was a small marble block with a carving on the front. As we stepped closer, we could see the front piece was an intricately constructed mosaic of a coat of arms. On the bottom section was the name Sarria, also in mosaic.

If we had been in a big hurry, just glancing as we walked by, we would have missed the intricate mosaic in this monument. It was an auspicious start to our Camino journey.

Today's hike was 22.7 km (14.1 miles) to Portomarin, just a little longer than the 13.1-mile half marathons we each had completed in around 4 hours earlier this year. So, with our planned comfortable pace of 2 miles an hour, we would arrive at our destination in 8 hours or so.

We kept our eyes out for yellow arrows and were soon rewarded with a small sign that guided us off the road onto a narrow, rocky trail. We had read that the first portion of today's hike would be a gradual climb of 150 meters, about 500 feet. Since we had supplemented our training in flat Florida by climbing steps at bridges and the St. Augustine Lighthouse, this elevation change didn't sound too daunting.

But even with all our training, we were out of breath after 20 minutes. We found a shady spot to rest and took a few more pictures. By now the trail had filled with other hikers, many of them puffing and struggling as they trudged on by. We were still getting our trail legs.

After climbing that first hill, we settled into a smooth and comfortable hiking rhythm, recognizing many sights from YouTube videos and Facebook posts. There was the giant stone bridge archway, the short stone wall along gravel paths, the lushly canopied forest trails.

After our struggle on the first hill, we had another surprise when we passed another marker. "Wait a minute," I said. "I thought it was 100 km from Sarria to Santiago, but there are still three digits in front of the decimal point." I put on my glasses and bent down to read the little km plate. It showed 112 km. That didn't make sense. We'd been hiking for almost an hour.

Jane whipped out her guidebook. "Well, what do you know. We had been so focused on the requirement to hike *at least* 100 km, we never added up the distance for our entire trek or checked the actual distance from Sarria." We all burst out laughing. So, our actual hike would end up being around 115 km, 72 miles instead of 62 miles. Even better.

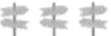

After a few miles, we stopped at a café so Jane and Cathy could take a bathroom break. I stood by the wall on the side of the path, drinking water and doing a few stretches and poses.

A woman walked up behind me. "Praying?" she asked.

"Nope, Tai Chi," I smiled.

"Nice!" She laughed. "Good idea. I guess even Tai Chi can be spiritual. Carry on."

When she mentioned the word "spiritual," it dawned on me I was still feeling anxious, wondering how I'd do, worrying about my feet. I remembered the serenity I felt in my classes back home as I engaged in a moving meditation, listening to Wil chant, "relax, relax, relax." *I should be able to capture that same spirit here surrounded by all this beauty.* That *angelic* woman reminded me to stop, take a deep breath, and calm the lurking chaos in my brain.

We trained for this trip with a focus on stamina until we were able to comfortably walk 5-6 miles a day for several days in a row. Our 2-mile-an-hour pace allowed plenty of time to take pictures, pause, and appreciate unusual sights. On our own. Nothing to prove. No need to rush. We walked slower than most others and happily stepped aside to let people pass when the trail tapered. Even when the trail got crowded, it seemed peaceful.

The trail would be totally quiet, then suddenly we'd be surrounded by a chorus of clomping boots and *"Buen Camino"* chants. We had read about the people and their reasons for hiking the Camino de Santiago. Some are devout. Others hope to find direction or tap into a hidden source of strength, a test of endurance. Many come to heal or to do homage to those they had lost.

The full length of 500 miles calls to many, just like the entire length of the Appalachian Trail calls to others, or how the full length of the ODH called to me. The shorter length of 115 km (72 miles) offered us an opportunity to accomplish a physical feat that would have been illusive and unobtainable if we had fixated on the entire 500 miles.

"Have you noticed the rock walls?" I asked Cathy. "They're made of fieldstone, rocks they had to dig up out of the fields so they could farm. I can't imagine all the work it must have taken. Then they probably looked at all those piles of rocks and said, 'Oh what the heck, let's build some walls and houses, maybe even a few bridges.'"

Cathy laughed. "Very good description, Sandi. Stand there so I can take a picture of you by the wall."

We looked ahead and spotted little round tables clustered just off the trail and decided to stop for lunch. I stamped my passport. This *cello* was red with an outline of a plump loaf of bread.

We walked by more fieldstone walls, through meadows, over small rock bridges, and musical bubbling brooks. We came around a corner and heard a different song. In the middle of nowhere, standing by a shade tree was a young man dressed in the medieval pilgrim costume: red hat and pants, white blouse, decorated vest. He was playing a flute-like instrument. The music was not familiar but sweetly lyrical, echoing the landscape. We stopped to listen. I saw a container on the ground holding money and quickly realized this was a photo op too good to pass by. "Jane, do you want to have your picture taken with him?"

"Oh yes!" We listened to more of his beautiful music, tossed coins in his hat, exchanged "*Gracias*!" with him and continued walking.

About an hour later, when the sun started blazing, we were delighted to find a small ramada with stone benches where we could sit in the shade and sip some water. An older man walked by pulling his backpack on a cart. "Are you selling sandwiches?" he called out. We laughed, he waved, and walked on.

When we met up with him about 30 minutes later as we climbed a short, steep hill, he was dragging. "I had planned to go to Santiago, but I decided to call it quits at the next town. I'm 78 years old and proud I walked an entire day on the Camino, but one day is enough for me. I'm tired. I've had enough of nature. I want to get back to Barcelona with people and cafes and buildings."

There it was! Plan B. He hiked the Camino *his way.*

We had about three miles left. Totally alone on the trail. The towns and cafes had evaporated. "I wonder what happened to all the people," Jane said.

Cathy responded, "I remember one of the other women I met on the train said she was planning to hike just 11 km (6.8 miles) today. People who hike this trail have lots of options to go as far as they want each day. I noticed *casas* and *albergues* (Spanish for hostel) in almost every town we walked through, so maybe many people have already stopped for the night."

We walked downhill for two miles, finally saw the bridge to Portomarin, and noticed a steep flight of stairs leading up to the town. We groaned but had to laugh. There were only about 50 steps, a piece of cake in terms of our training. Just not our favorite thing at the end of the day. Even this large block staircase was ancient and beautiful.

We arrived at Hotel Ferramenteiro, a lovely structure built into the mountainside. The lobby had a large plate glass window across the entire back wall with a spectacular view of the valley below. Our rooms were neat, narrow, sparse, and hot. "Just open your windows. The evening breeze will cool things down very soon," offered the friendly desk clerk. "Breakfast will open at 7:30. And you can get your *cellos* then."

We agreed to meet back in the lobby at 5:30. I went to my room, took off my socks and shoes, and did a little physical assessment. My feet felt fine! I'm sure the poles were a big help. No blisters or hot spots, no other aches or pains. I propped up my feet on the bed and called Arnie. We were just five hours ahead so my end-of-hike calls would work out perfect for us, especially since every lodge had Wi-Fi.

"Hi, hon," Arnie answered. "How are you? How was your first day on the trail?"

"I'm fine. The trail was beautiful, more than I ever dreamed it would be. How are you?"

"I'm great. I had a good morning. Got out on my bike and am just getting ready to eat lunch."

"Super. It looks like this is the best time to chat each day whenever we arrive from the day's hike. I'm thinking about leaving a little early tomorrow morning to beat the heat. I'll text you when I leave. You probably won't hear much from me during the day."

"That's fine. Just be careful and have fun. I'm glad it's working out so well for you. Please tell Jane and Cathy hi for me. Love you."

"Thanks, hon, I will. Love you."

I was concerned about Day Two, the longest hike of our trek, 24.6 km (15.3 miles), most of it uphill. Temperatures were forecasted in the 90s. I knew I could do it, but the heat would make it harder for me. I would be much slower. Morning is my best time and I wanted to get as many miles in as I could before the afternoon sun hit. Cathy and Jane wanted to wait for the 7:30 breakfast so we might not get started until 8:30. If I left early, I could get almost two hours of hiking in before full daylight. I made my decision and asked the desk clerk to stamp my passport.

Day Two

I got up at 5:00, drank two *café con leches* from the lobby vending machine, ate a few granola bars, and hit the trail at 6:00. Just a little before daybreak. I was alone at first, but within minutes, three other hikers came up in front of me from a side street. A woman named Peggy caught up with me from behind. It was nice to have someone else to confirm we were on the right path, especially when we passed one little fork with no visible arrow.

We walked together for about 25 minutes, sharing our stories. Then she headed off at a faster pace. It was still darkish and foggy with lovely night sounds, but the trail was getting easier to follow. All of it was a little eerie and incredibly beautiful. The incline was gradual. I celebrated every hour in this comfortable cool as I slowly increased my pace, trying to beat the heat: 7:00 am, 2.5 miles; 8:00 am, 4.75 miles.

The trail opened wide on top of a hill with just a few trees lining the path. A celestial glow preceded the full sun, creating a moment of quiet beauty that gently reminded me to stop and savor this moment. To enjoy this awesome journey.

Fifteen minutes later, the path narrowed and turned a corner. Now I was walking between two fieldstone walls with farmland on either side. And then, a fork in the path with yellow arrows going opposite ways. After a moment of panic, I remembered reading in the guidebook last night that I would have a choice. I could turn right and stay on the main path that bordered a busy, noisy road. Or I could turn left and take a slight detour that the guidebook described as bucolic and beautiful.

The few hikers ahead of me all turned right toward the road. If I took the detour, I'd be alone, which made me a little nervous. And it might take a little longer. I pondered another minute. *I may never pass this way again, so I'll take the path less traveled. I'm pretty sure Frost would be proud.* And so I turned left into another opportunity to approach this trek *my way*.

The muddy trail passed by an empty field with lumps of dirt and old equipment sitting around. Some were tipped over, all stuck in mud and glowing in the morning sun. The trail angled right, gradually widened, and turned into a cobblestone path leading to a small village with buildings constructed of small dark stones. When I came to a crossroad and couldn't see any arrows, I stopped. *I made a big mistake and now I'm lost.*

A woman's voice came up behind me. "You didn't make a mistake. You made the right choice. The guidebook says to turn right to the ancient church and a café; then you will see the arrows." She went on ahead of me and turned right. I followed. She was carrying a heavy backpack and in a hurry. After taking a few pictures of the church, she turned and waved *Buen Camino*, and took off. I never even learned her name, so I decided to call her *trail angel* and marveled at another chance encounter with a total stranger.

I walked into a beautiful old parlor by the café and stamped my passport with another unique *cello*, a blue outline of a km marker, K82 (51 miles), a scallop shell with the name, location, and telephone number of *Casa Garcia*. I stepped out, saw the yellow arrows and was soon back on the path. After another mile, my fortuitous fork converged with the main route crowded with other hikers.

Around 11:30, I arrived at the highest point on the trail. A tall, slender woman with wild curly hair stood straight, hands on her hips, surveying the scenery. We introduced ourselves. She took my picture, and we shared our stories. Regina had traveled here from Germany. This was the third and final portion of her 500+ mile *Camino de Santiago* hike that she had split over three years. Since Regina still worked full-time, this was the only way she could fit the entire Camino into her annual two-week vacation schedule. "I'm going to stay here a while longer, Sandi," she said as I turned to go. "I want to savor this high point on today's hike. You helped make this stop even more memorable. Perhaps we will see each other again. *Buen Camino*."

"You did the same for me," I said. "Thank you, and *Buen Camino*."

The summit climb was over. It was downhill, but the heat finally caught up with me. I stopped at another café around 1:00. I sat and drank juice, ordered some lunch, and relaxed, considering my morning. I met three fellow hikers: Peggy, *trail angel*, and Regina. The hosts in *Casa Garcia* and in this café were kind and generous. The piece of *Spanish Omelette* he brought out to my table was so big, I wrapped up half and stuffed it in my backpack. I had set out early to avoid the heat and found myself encountering multiple rays of human warmth.

Around 2:30, I was ready for another break. As I sat in the patio of the cafe, drinking coffee and munching on a piece of my leftover *Spanish Omelette*, Jane and Cathy walked into the courtyard. We celebrated our reunion, got our stamps, and hit the trail.

We stopped again at 3:30 for shade, a quick, refreshing lemonade, and another stamp. Most of the *cellos* so far looked topical, usually of monuments or costumed pilgrims. But this one was designed with four ants. There had to be some story. Then Jane looked down the trail and pointed out a set of giant ant sculptures just beyond the umbrella-covered tables. Four of them. Of course.

As we admired the ants and took pictures, I thought, *If I had still been walking alone, exhausted at this point with my eyes glued on the trail, I might have missed these captivating sculptures. Leave it to Jane to notice them.*

Soon we were trudging more than hiking and quite happy that we had just two km (1.2 miles) left. Cathy and I plopped down on a rock. Jane went into a gas station to check our route and found out it was two *miles* not km's. We moaned and muttered, then looked around, found a bench at a bus stop, sat down, and started to laugh. We didn't even have the energy to take a selfie. Nobody came by who could take our picture. So we just decided we would have to keep this picture in our minds. This picture of three bedraggled old ladies sitting together on a bench waiting for the bus that never came.

"Two more miles? Well, we can sit here waiting for a bus from somewhere going somewhere else, or never coming at all. Or we can keep walking," said Jane.

We finally slogged into Palas de Rei at 4:30, stepping into a beautiful stone courtyard. We climbed down a short staircase to the main road and things immediately looked up. We quickly found our hotel, grabbed our bags from the lobby, and went to our rooms to freshen up and rest a bit before dinner.

And best of all I could call Arnie and let him know how my early start to this longest day had worked out perfectly.

Days Three and Four

Palas De Rei to Melide was one of our shorter days. Our travel company had offered the option of combining the two shorter hikes on days three and four into one long day of hiking, but we were happy to break it up into nine miles today and eight miles tomorrow. We did not have to rush through our trip to scurry back to work and we were more than ready for a few shorter days.

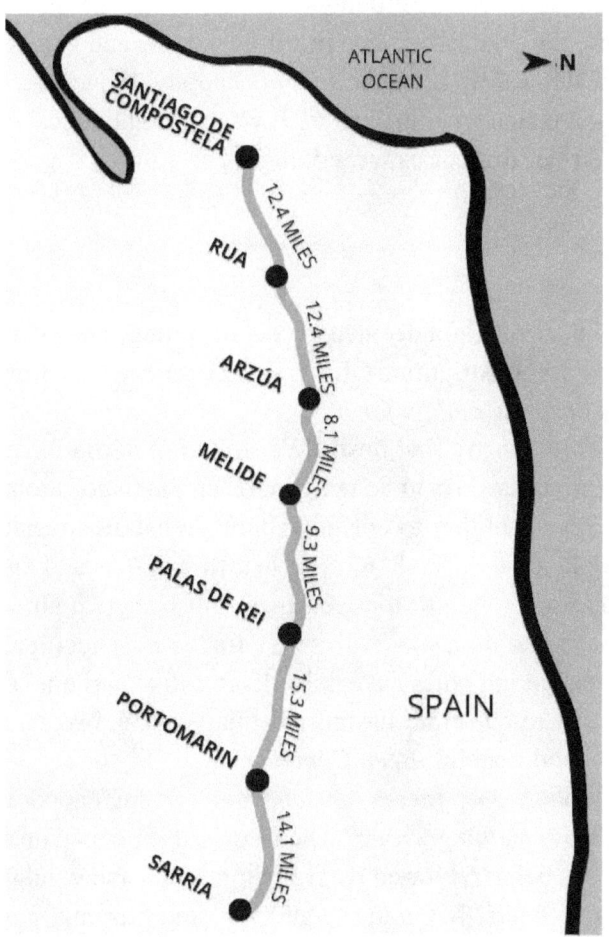

Later that day, we saw old people! As we ate our lunch under a café ramada, a sea of 25 people, all our age, all wearing blue scarves, flowed off the trail and splashed into the patio. Later, while we waited in line for our *cellos,* we chatted with Annette, the leader. "For many years, our school sponsored Camino de

Santiago treks for our graduating seniors," she said. "A few years ago, we decided to include their grandparents for a portion of the hike. The children hike with their peers at a faster pace, able to tour more places along the trail, then both groups get back together at Santiago. We are delighted to see the unique bond this experience creates between the grandparents and grandchildren."

After a few more hours, we happily arrived at our hotel, Pension Berenguela in Melide. It was getting hotter. I checked in with Arnie. Both of us were doing well.

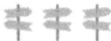

That evening, I decided to take the plunge and post an update in the Facebook Camino Group. *Just introduce your story, include a few pictures, and go for it.*

This was my first post: "We started in Sarria three days ago and have three days to go until we reach Santiago, a total of about 75 miles according to our guidebook. What an adventure for us three old ladies: 75, 68, 67. I have artificial hips and knees, atrial fib, and severely arthritic feet. I was most worried about my feet, but have had no issues with stress fractures, tendonitis, not even blisters. Hiking poles have helped! This hike was one of the ways I wanted to celebrate turning 75 this year, and so far, so good! Happy and grateful. *Buen Camino!*"

I took a deep breath, hit *send*, and nothing happened. *Oh no! Did I do something wrong?* Then a message popped up saying my post was being reviewed by group managers and would be posted in a few hours. My mind would not stop buzzing. I tossed and turned, finally settled in for a few hours of deep sleep.

The next morning, I opened Facebook to see if my message had been posted and was stunned. It was there along with more than 300 likes and 50 comments, many saying *"Buen Camino"* or "Congratulations." But there were also more heart-warming comments. "You have motivated me. I have two artificial knees and asthma and plan on doing it next spring when I'm 73. Any tips on how you prepared?" Someone else said: "Inspired me! I'm 67 and was wondering if I could do it in the next couple of years. Now I think I might go for it."

I responded to as many questions as I could, especially those asking for tips with the promise I'd provide more detail after I got home. *What a nice surprise. Maybe my Camino tale can make a difference.* It motivated me to continue posting updates. I realized that telling my story could be a new purpose in my life. Another way to influence and inspire.

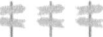

On Day 4, we hiked from Melide to Arzua, our second short day. We were at the halfway point in our trek. Three days in, three days to go. Each day brought more confidence and collegiality.

We three are different people, but united in our passion of action travel and growing appreciation of each other. I wasn't sure if Cathy and Jane were seeking something specific on this hike, but I knew Cathy well enough to understand she approaches every day in a spirit of gratitude, especially with her liver transplant. And Jane? She loves to travel, so I guessed she was seeking a new tourist experience. Then today, I learned something else.

After hiking through several shallow river valleys, the path smoothed out through forests of giant oaks, then eucalyptus and pine. We turned at the next yellow arrow and saw a little sign directing us to a small chapel for a *cello*. Jane went in first and was standing in line waiting for the priest to stamp her passport when I called her name. She turned and flashed one of her happiest smiles for a photo.

The slender priest wore grey slacks, a navy zipper sweater over a blue plaid shirt, and was sitting at a small wooden table. He slowly stamped each passport, wrote the date, and latched eyes with each of us. The chapel was dark and inviting. His table was perched on the stone floor in front of an altar with a crucifix on one side and a statue of a pilgrim on the other. Cathy and I left some money in the little basket on the priest's table and stepped outside to wait for Jane.

She came out a few minutes later. "I have a habit of lighting a candle on every trip for my mom, who is in a nursing home. This small church spoke to me, so that's where I chose to light her candle, rather than the big cathedral at the end."

Jane turned quickly to head on, followed by Cathy. But I stood still for just a moment. Her story touched my heart. I learned a bit more about Jane's spiritual journey. I thought about my own mom and remembered that I had carried a few painted rocks with me. I took the one with a heart and placed it on the next km marker we passed. Mom would have loved this hike.

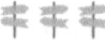

Since I had not slept well the night before, I was so tired that at our first coffee stop I stamped my hand instead of my passport! But that wasn't the craziest thing I did on Day 4. I saved that for the end of the day's hike.

We made our way across an ancient bridge with a slight peak over three arches and into Arzua. As we walked along the main street for what seemed like miles, Jane suddenly stopped and checked her map. "I think we missed our hotel. We may have to backtrack," she said.

"I need to sit and drink something," I said as we passed by a café. "Let's stop here and maybe you can ask someone." I sat on a bench, set down my gear, and drank some water.

Jane asked the woman standing at the café entrance for directions to our hotel. "Oh no, you didn't miss it," the woman said. "Your hotel is just three blocks ahead. On the right."

I jumped up. We walked with new energy and quickly arrived at the hotel. The man at the front desk looked very concerned.

"You forgot something," he said. "You have to go back."

"Oh no, is our luggage lost?" Jane asked. "Did we put it in the wrong place back in Melide?"

"No, you have to go back," he said. Then he looked at me, "Are you Sandra? You forgot something." Then my stomach dropped. My heart started pounding. I didn't have my backpack! I scolded myself. *All my medicine, supplies, journal, essentials. How could I have done this? Where did I forget it? How many miles back? What have I done?*

When he saw my look of terror, he gave us our room keys. "Your luggage is in the hall," he said. "Take your bags to your room and I'll go back and pick up your backpack and bring it to you."

I walked to my room frantic with confusion. *How did he know my name? How far back would he have to go?* Then I remembered. It was back at the café where we stopped to get directions. I was so tired I just jumped up when we found out the hotel was nearby and completely forgot my backpack. Thank goodness it was just a few blocks and not miles away. I grabbed some money out of my pocket and sat on the bed facing my open door.

In just a few minutes, Gabriel came with my backpack and extended his hand. I had ten euros and reached out to give it to him. He shook his head. "No. no. I don't want your money," he said, smiling.

"I have to give you something for your trouble," I insisted.

He pulled back his hand. "No, no you don't. I'm the manager and we take care of our guests." Then he extended his hand again. We shook hands, both of us with big smiles and full hearts.

It turns out that the lady who gave Jane directions remembered what hotel we were going to. She noticed my backpack on the bench and saw my ID tag. She called our hotel and notified Gabriel at the front desk. Now this was Camino magic! Later that evening, when we went to the front desk to get our passports stamped, Gabriel walked around the corner, stood close, looked me straight in the eye, and flashed that kind and beautiful smile. "From now on, Sandra, remember your backpack." Sound guidance from another *trail angel*.

Day Four ended with my growing realization that the Camino was much more than mere miles from Sarria to Santiago. More than just pushing my body. I was moving from simply seeing to being. Trail magic was creating a force in me, migrating from physical to spiritual.

Day Five

We left before breakfast, figuring we'd grab something at the first café along the way. It was going to be another hot day and all three of us wanted to hike as far as we could before the full sun hit. On the way out of town, we walked by an ancient cemetery filled with tall stone structures. We felt ourselves being drawn in for just a few minutes to walk along narrow paths, reading the names and dates of those who passed. We stepped back on the trail and started up an incline. Oh, morning glory! Our early start was rewarded by a brilliant sunrise just as we crested the hill.

Rolling hills surrounded by forests and sunlit fields looked like impressionist paintings. Someone called my name. It was Regina, the lovely woman I met at the summit on Day Two who had split her Camino journey into three years. I wanted to hug her but felt a little awkward. I barely knew her. So I asked if we could have our picture taken together and looped my arm around her waist for the photo. She did the same and asked Jane to take a picture with her camera too. She sped on ahead. "I hope to see you at the end."

This portion of the hike took us through small towns with little sights that called out for photo collages. Without even planning a strategy, we each focused on a different theme.

Jane captured yellow arrows painted on walls, outlined in

rocks along the path, etched in bricks, embedded in mosaics surrounding doors. Cathy had been captivated early on by the high-rising corn cribs. These big rectangle boxes stood on long narrow wooden stilts, looking like sentries along the trail in almost every plot of farmland we passed.

I took pictures of flowers, especially those artfully planted along the paths. One wall was festooned with yellow shelves holding shoes and boots that served as planters. No shoe was the same; neither were the flowers. An array of succulents, purple petunias, yellow mums, pink impatiens, bright green ivy. A large boot on the ground held a light-green vine and boasted a bright yellow arrow painted across its toe. That boot earned a photo in both my and Jane's collages. Other flowers sprouted out of holes between the stones in the wall.

We passed by a tiny *albergues* built of small rocks with a black slate roof. Along the wall was a petite alcove altar surrounded by pots of multi-colored flowers. A hand-painted sign offered "Free Hugs!" More towns, more flowers, arrows, and tiny decorative corn cribs, dramatically different than our first days on the trail.

Since we had started earlier that morning, we arrived at our casa in time for lunch in a tree-shaded garden. It was a beautiful spot to spend our last day on the trail before hiking to Santiago tomorrow.

Over lunch we relaxed, enjoying the scenery, chatting with other hikers each with their own story. Jane and Cathy decided to walk around the town and see if they could find a good place for dinner. For the first time during our hike, I decided to play the age card. "I would love to join you, but I'm too tired. I need to sit, write a few notes in my journal, and rest."

"Enjoy yourself. You're entitled. One of my fondest dreams is that I can be as active as you when I'm 75," said Jane.

I sat under the trees, writing in my journal, reading, and enjoying the peace. I settled into a quiet reverie. *This trek ended up being much more than I expected. Camino spirit and magic grew each day, each encounter, each experience, and each interaction among the three of us.*

Cathy was bubbling when they returned. "Sandi, we didn't see many places to eat but we got to tour a brand new *albergue*. You would have loved seeing it."

"Oh, you're right! Darn it. I'm sorry I missed it."

Cathy responded with her usual thoughtful perspective, "Well, remember, we missed that beautiful little village you visited when you took that detour on Day Two. We turned right and missed that. We just can't do it all, and I have to tell you, you look mighty content sitting in this beautiful spot."

"The food is so good here," Jane said, "why don't we eat in their indoor restaurant tonight?" It was the perfect place to spend our last dinner on the trail. Jane flirted with the chef who served us, teasing him about his name. "Nacho? Do you know what a nacho is in the United States?"

He laughed. "Of course, I do. My name is Ignacio, shortened to Nacho. And it's just a coincidence that I became a chef and nachos are a fun food in America." We all burst out laughing. He was charming, cheerful, very handsome, and having a great time bantering with Jane.

There were just a few others in the restaurant since it was still early, so we took our time enjoying our meal, even ordering dessert for our final fling. "Remember to put your ponchos in your backpacks," Cathy reminded us. "Rain is forecasted, and it's supposed to be cooler."

"It might be nice to have some different weather as long as it doesn't rain too hard," I said. "I have mixed feelings about tomorrow being our last day. What about you two?"

"I'm ready to be done, but I will miss this trail and our fun times together," Jane admitted. "I'm excited about touring the cathedral in Santiago, also getting our certificates. Did you know they even write our names in Latin? I saw some pictures on

Facebook. They're beautiful. If we get there early enough, maybe we can get them tomorrow. I read there are usually long lines, but maybe we'll get lucky."

"Same," said Cathy. "I'm ready to stop walking, but I don't want this journey and our time together to end."

"Sandi, get some wine tonight," Cathy insisted. "We need a toast." We poured the wine, clinked our glasses, and toasted to our last night on the trail. *Buen Camino!*

Day Six

Morning broke clear and sunny, our final day on the Camino. We stepped back on the trail, anxious and excited. We were intimidated by the final steep incline described in our guidebook as "a long slog," so we braced ourselves for achy legs. But it never happened. We climbed at a brisk pace and felt fine. Well, what do you know? We had already hiked more than 65 miles in five days. Our bodies had acclimated. Even though this climb was steeper than our initial climb on Day 1, we were stronger.

The farther we walked, the more crowded the path became. "The guidebook said most of the other Camino trails will converge today so we'll probably have lots of company," Jane said. The calm peace of ambling hikers gave way to a fast, even frantic pace. A few were even jogging as we heard more calls of "coming through!" Easy to understand the need for speed as hikers neared the end, especially those who had been on the trail for weeks, even months.

Our excitement increased as the distance to Santiago decreased. The crowds surged forward, and we stepped off the main trail. First, we hiked up Monte do Gozo to the enormous commemorative Pope Juan Pablo II monument. Then, continuing off the beaten path, we climbed a second hill to reach the statue of two 12-foot-high pilgrims pointing to Santiago. This statue was majestic. Because we had not hiked the entire 500+ miles of the

Camino, we had missed seeing many of the monuments that appeared in *The Way*. We could not and would not miss this one.

We were completely alone. For just a moment, our world stood still. It started to sprinkle, but we stayed, letting this moment soak in. When our hearts were full and our ponchos drenched, we headed back down to the nearly empty trail.

The path grew wider, monuments became more plentiful, and kilometer markers grew smaller as we entered Santiago. Our time on the Camino ended abruptly as we crossed a busy street, walked down a hill, and saw our first traffic light.

We relied more on the map now, but mostly we just looked for tired backpackers and followed them. The crowds thinned. We kept losing our way, stopping at street corners, not sure which way to turn. "Well, Ivan was right about following the yellow arrows and not getting lost on the trail," Jane said. "But we forgot to ask him how to resume finding our way *without* the arrows. This is crazy!"

We turned a few more corners and finally saw the tunnel. "Please go ahead. I want to wait here for just a few minutes. I'll find you in the square," I said to Cathy and Jane. I love endings as much as beginnings and did not want to rush these final steps to the finish line. I stopped and let this moment seep in. When there was a break in the crowd, I stepped forward. Just then the Cathedral bells started chiming. I waited until the tolling stopped, the sound waves settled, and my breathing slowed.

As I walked down the gentle slope of the tunnel, I heard more music. It was a beautiful melody like the one we heard on the trail our first day. This time it came from a bagpipe! The musician sat off to the side at the bottom. Her music reverberated throughout the small tunnel core. I paused to soak in another musical moment, then walked over. "*Gracias*," I said and dropped some coins into her open case.

I proceeded out the tunnel and into Cathedral Square. The air was misting and magical as I walked into the square and turned to look up at the tall spires of the Santiago Cathedral. After hearing the chimes and the bagpipe, I fully expected a choir to start singing. I waited. Nope. Didn't happen. So I simply enjoyed the faint chorus of Leonard Cohen singing *Hallelujah* in my head.

I found Cathy and Jane and we headed to the Pilgrim Office to get our *Compostela* today. After a longish wait in line, I stepped up to a counter and saw an elderly lady with a warm smile and blue eyes sitting at a low table. She reminded me of Jane Goodall. "May I please see your passport ID and your Camino passport? Where did you start your journey?"

"Sarria," I responded as I proudly handed her my two passports.

"Oh, so you hiked from Sarria. That's 115 kilometers. Congratulations. You hiked far enough to earn the *Compostela*. Now I'll check your stamps," she explained as she opened my Camino passport. She thoroughly reviewed each page, pointing to each stamp with her pen, counting stamps, making sure there were at least two for each day. "Okay, good," she looked up and smiled. "Now there is one final question."

Her smile turned serious. Her eyes probing. "Why did you make this pilgrimage?" she asked as she pointed to three lines with a little box behind each. She picked up her pen poised to check one of those boxes. "Are you a tourist? Was this a physical challenge? Or was it spiritual?" Then she looked up at me, her blue eyes clear and focused as she waited for my answer.

"Well, I began with several goals, including hiking this trail as a tourist and for the physical challenge."

She tilted her head, kept looking at me, giving me the time to think, not moving her pen.

"But somewhere along the trail, the hike turned into a pilgrimage for me. It became more spiritual," I said.

Then she positioned her pen over the little box behind spiritual. "So it's spiritual, right?" She smiled as she checked the box. "I thought so."

I had qualified for my certificate. She placed a final stamp in my Camino passport, carefully transcribed my name in English on one document and in Latin on the other, *Alexandram Richmond*, and handed my documents to me, looking genuinely proud. From one old woman to another, she reached up her hand to shake mine. "Congratulations, Sandra. I am very happy for you."

The memory of that moment will remain long after my certificate gets lost.

I walked through the door back out to the street. Cathy and Jane stood holding their certificates, smiling, waiting for me. We high-fived each other. "It's official. We made it. We're certified."

While Cathy and Jane shopped for souvenirs, I headed back to the tunnel to take a few pictures. On my way I saw Regina. "Sandi? I hoped I'd get to see you one more time. We made it!" She said with a big smile. I walked up and there was no hesitancy this time. We wrapped each other in a bear hug. She hung on a little longer.

"Congratulations, Regina! It took three years for you to get here. You must be overwhelmed with joy."

She nodded. "I am. Thank you for being here to celebrate with me. Congratulations to you too, Sandi. I'm happy for both of us."

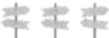

Later, during a phone call with Rachel, I shared one of my favorite quotes from John Brierly's *Camino Guidebook*:

To try is to risk failure. But risks must be taken. Because the greatest hazard in life is to risk nothing.

The people who risk nothing may avoid suffering and sorrow. But they cannot learn, feel, change, grow or really live.

And then, this is crazy. I started to cry when I read the final line:

Only a person who risks is truly free.

"Where did that come from?" I gasped.

Rachel said after a pause. "Maybe this was a bigger deal than you realized."

"Maybe so," I said. "I don't think I really acknowledged how scared I was, wondering if my body would really hold up for six whole days. This distance was almost four times as long as the Inca Trail and I am three years older."

Rachel listened quietly.

"I guess I got choked up because I had been scared, but I think the bigger reason may be because I was overjoyed everything worked out so well."

I paused. "When I first started, the notion of *Camino magic* just sounded too cliché for me. But there *was* magic. In the scenery. The other hikers. The people who provided food and lodging. In my relationship with Cathy and Jane. Even my love for Dad who encouraged me every day, every way, every call. So, you're right, hon. It was a bigger deal than I imagined, but more in terms of goodness than in difficulty."

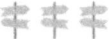

During this trip, I had become more trail-and-trip-smart, filled to the brim with new courage and confidence. My body and soul were infused with a new sense of strength and purpose. It was more than life changing. It was life affirming that I was headed in the right direction, on the right path, and in the right way. My way.

CHAPTER 15

Taking One Step Forward

It was June, and I was walking back into Dr. Mendez's office just about a year after she and I had faced-off with each other about all my walking. Dr. Mendez swooped in, carrying notes, smiling. "Hi, Sandi. Tell me what's going on."

I told her my story. "During the last few months when I'm walking without my hiking poles, my left foot gets weak, drifts over and hits my right foot, sometimes almost tripping me." In a burst of wishful thinking, I offer, "I think it might be my orthotics."

"Okay," she said. "Sit up on the table." She probed and asked questions as she went through the usual foot-strength drill. She pressed her hand down hard on top of my foot. "Push up against my hand as hard as you can." I did it easily.

She kept pushing and testing both feet, shaking her head. "I thought you might have *drop foot*, but your feet seem way too strong for that. Your left foot is a little weaker than your right, but both are pretty strong. Are you sure you don't have any back pain?"

"Yes, I'm sure. My feet hurt a little after I walk, but everything else is fine."

"I guess we just have to start ruling things out so we can figure out what's going on," she finally concluded. "You need to get a CT scan. An MRI would be better, but you can't have that because of your bladder inter-stem implant. And you should go to a podiatrist. We will figure this out. I know how important this is for you, and we will make sure you can continue walking."

She remembered how important walking was to me! We both had traveled a long way this past year.

A week after my CT scan, Dr. Mendez called, sounding unusually subdued. "The scan shows you have advanced spinal canal stenosis, so we need to talk about next steps. You need another scan with dye, but that would be handled by a neurosurgeon. Please come in so I can show you what's going on."

Advanced spinal canal stenosis? How could I go from a drifting left foot to a spinal issue? I tried to tell myself not to panic, at least not until I could learn what was going on. But I couldn't sleep that night. Back problems scare the heck out of me.

I came in the next day. The nurse ushered me to her office, asked me a few questions. "Doctor will be right in."

Dr. Mendez walked in, no swooping this time. She locked eyes with me as always, but her eyebrows were wrinkled with concern, even sadness. After a brief pause, she opened her computer. "Sandi, let me show you what's going on." She pointed to an X-ray. "This is a scan of your lower back. As we go down toward your tailbone to L4 and L5, there is significant narrowing of your spinal column. This lumbar narrowing is an issue."

She turned away from the screen. "As I told you on the phone, you will need more tests and should be under the care of a neurosurgeon. It's hard to get in, so we've already called Mayo Clinic in Jacksonville and they have started processing your paperwork. This does not necessarily mean you need surgery, but you definitely need more diagnostic tests."

When I told her I was walking longer and harder, she perked up and gave me a big smile. "You're doing your own PT! Keep it up. You can't hurt yourself and you're getting stronger."

The irony was not lost on me that she had told me last year to stop walking so much. But this was a different time, different issue, different concern. Bless her caring heart. She knew now that walking and staying active were the *best* things I could do mentally and physically.

I had expected this summer to provide a break in big events with some downtime to relax, renew, and then ramp up my training for the Grand Canyon. Instead, it ended up with lots of unanticipated twists. At this point I had no idea how many hills I'd have to climb before even getting to the canyon, much less hiking it. But I was determined to keep training hard and heading in that direction.

I continued to chat with myself during my walks, making sure I used my hiking poles since I was still unsteady. I listened to the birds singing, leaves rustling, and waves splashing from the boat wakes on the Intracoastal Waterway. Those sounds soothed me. Most of the time, my self-talk did the same.

The day after my appointment with Dr. Mendez, I gave myself lots of encouragement. "You are walking with no pain on a beautiful trail, getting stronger with every step. Your spine will be okay. You are okay. Enjoy this walk. Don't worry. Be happy. Just keep moving." My walking meditation quickly helped me get high on gratitude.

But soon I plunged into a deep chasm.

It was time to wrap up our Grand Canyon travel plans. A few days later, I opened the file, pulled out my North Rim confirmation email, and looked closely at the dates. My heart dropped. The usually calm voice in my head started wailing. The print on the copy of my North Rim lodging reservation was tiny, so I squinted, rubbing my eyes. I had made North Rim lodging reservations for 2018, not 2019. For *last* year, not *this* year!

How could I have done this? My heart was pounding. I could barely breathe. I frantically pulled up the website to search for my 2019 reservations. Nothing. The date had passed. I had made the reservations for the right days and wrong year.

So here I was in July 2019 with no North Rim reservations. Our trip was ruined!

But then I began to negotiate with myself. *Maybe it's for the best, especially since Rachel will be recovering from her Ironman event. Maybe this is a sign. But I don't believe in signs. I should just accept reality. We can still travel to the canyon, take a shorter hike, allow more time for Rachel to rest and heal and for me to adjust to time zone change and elevation. Accept and adjust.*

These options seemed reasonable. But my heart was breaking. There was a good chance this would be my final opportunity to do a one-day rim-to-rim. And I blew it.

I sat back in my desk chair and gazed at the tree outside my office window, waiting for the fog to clear. Eventually my perspective changed. *Nope, I want and need to do the rim-to-rim, nothing else. No Plan B. I need my rocking chair memory. There has to be a way. I have to find a way. No, we have to find a way. I'll call Rachel, but first I'll talk to Arnie. He will give me perspective and a path forward. I don't have to figure this out on my own.*

Arnie calmed me down after a little sigh. "Go ahead and make your other arrangements, and we'll just keep checking to see if a North Rim reservation opens up. We have two months!"

I needed to call Rachel, hating to add to her pressure since she was training hard with Rob for their Ironman event in Cambridge, Maryland. Yes, Rachel was doing an Ironman the day before our scheduled flight to Arizona. She was also helping her younger son Andrew get everything together for starting college in the fall. And helping her older son Jonathan with his training and preparation for going to Army Basic Training.

I took a big breath. Then one more. "Hi, hon. I think I get the reward for doing the dumbest thing ever for any of our trips together. I was so proud of myself for making our North Rim reservations, but I made them for October 2, 2018!"

"Oh, Mom, I'm so sorry! I know how crazy that canyon reservation system is and I can see how easy that was to do. Please don't worry, we can find a way. Maybe we can get campground reservations on the North Rim and I can carry a light tent. We will make this work, whatever it takes!"

"Rachel, I know how important this is for you to be home with Jonathan before he leaves. Maybe we should wait until next year."

"No, we shouldn't. My schedule has gotten harder to manage and I do feel a little torn, but we can make this work. It means Rob, Andrew, and Jonathan can have some special time together while we're at the canyon. You know as well as I do we may never have this chance again. We have no idea what next year will bring."

Rachel paused. "I don't want you to use this as an excuse to stop trying to get reservations, but if we can't get reservations, we could even do a rim-to-rim-to-rim. We could hike over to the North Rim trailhead, rest, wrap up in our space blankets for a few hours on the North Rim, and then just turn around and hike back to the South Rim. We'd have to carry more food and some warm clothes, but we know the drill."

Resorting to a R2R2R made perfect sense. No, it didn't. It was insane. An absolutely crazy plan. But it did indicate the extent of Rachel's determination to make this work for me. This could easily be our last chance to take this hike together.

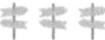

My Prolia injections had improved my bone strength and provided a huge boost of confidence. One of my biggest fears for this year was that one of my feet would break again. Foot issues had prevented me from doing this one-day rim-to-rim hike with Rachel three times before due to a stress fracture, a torn ligament, and tendonitis. And then, that other bone broke when I was walking slowly down the street with Arnie. I did not trust my feet. They had let me down too often.

But since I had started receiving Prolia injections in 2018, my feet had gotten stronger, worthy of renewed trust. They stood the test of the events I had already completed this year.

I drove into the hospital parking lot in a state of grace and joy. Before I left the car, I sat there for a few minutes basking in my bubble of gratitude. *I am lucky. I am privileged. I am grateful. My injection is administered in the cancer center. I'm getting ready to have a foot-saving Prolia injection in a room filled with people who are getting life-saving infusions.* Just walking into the waiting room reminded me of how fortunate I was in terms of my health. The other patients sat calmly, most of them chatting, smiling. They were warriors.

The nurse called me in from the waiting room. I noticed she was new and didn't have the usual warm smile that greeted me as we moved to the prep room to record my weight and check my blood-work results.

She looked at the computer, took a big breath, then flashed a big smile. "Good news! You don't have to get a shot today. You are free to go."

Of course, this was *not* good news. It wasn't remotely logical. I knew it was dangerous to simply stop this treatment without medical guidance. That bubble of joy I felt when I came in suddenly burst. Panic fogged my brain as I reached for my purse getting ready to leave. Then I heard a voice, my voice, calling through the fog. *Do not move. Stop and think. Calm down.* I crossed my arms gently, sat still, breathed deeply.

The nurse fidgeted, looking uncomfortable. A precious few minutes had passed. My brain fog had cleared. No more panic. Much more perspective. *Do I leave and try to fight this later? No, I don't. There's no way I'm leaving without my shot!*

I looked up at the anxious nurse. "This is *not* good news. It doesn't even make sense. When I started this series of shots, I was told I would get four shots over two years. Then a follow-up bone scan would determine progress and next steps. This would be shot #4 and my bone scan isn't even scheduled yet. What's going on? Why aren't you allowed to give me this shot?"

She slowly responded. "The front office told me there was a recent Medicare audit and you are no longer eligible for coverage. Your bone scan from 2017 showed you have osteopenia and Medicare only covers Prolia shots for those patients with osteoporosis."

Since my primary care doctor had just retired, I'd have to be my own advocate until I secured a new doctor. "This was the case when my previous doctor originally petitioned Medicare for coverage. Although my bone scan indicated osteopenia, I had incurred several fractures in my feet. She included all that information in her original referral notes. That's why these shots were approved in the first place."

The nurse checked her computer, read a little further, and blinked when she saw the notes I referred to. She nodded. "I need to go check with my supervisor. Please wait here."

The nurse returned. "They refiled your entire profile with Medicare and we'll trust they will cover this. Let's take you in for your shot."

Now I could get back to my training and not worry about my feet, just the heat and my spine.

Arnie came with me to my appointment at Mayo with neurosurgeon, Dr. Kingsley Abode, 38 years old with impressive credentials.

Whenever I encounter a new doctor, I make it a point to *dress for success.* I apply extra mascara to brighten my eyes and wear athletic clothes. As I've aged, I've learned that how I show up for that initial appointment is critical. My quality-of-life saver. I can't take the chance that I will be dismissed because of my birth date or artificial joints. I need to be seen as an athlete. Leaving nothing to chance, I even wore my Inca Trail T-shirt to this appointment.

I understand Medicare needs guidelines and standards, but

I'm concerned about an inherent ageism in the system that sometimes does not adequately support healthy, active seniors.

The door opened. Dr. Abode strode in, shook my hand, then Arnie's. He stepped over to the computer and picked up my Camino itinerary I had given to his nurse. His smile got bigger as he asked a few questions about my hike, nodding, clearly impressed.

He turned to the computer and reviewed the scan. His smile faded. It seemed like he was dealing with a bit of cognitive dissonance. He looked at me, then back at the scan.

"What does it say?" I asked.

He nodded. "I'll show you the results. I just need to test a few things first." Then he did all the same things Dr. Mendez did, pushing my feet, asking me to press back, calling out directions like a gentle drill sergeant. I did my best to comply, especially with my left foot. But I could tell I wasn't moving his hand as far as I was with my right foot. "You need some PT to build up the strength in your left foot," he said.

Dr. Abode finally turned back to the computer. "Okay, let me show you what's going on with your spine." He pointed to minor disk compression. "That's not an issue right now, somewhat normal for your age." Then he pointed to the lower part, L4-L5. "This is serious. At some point, this narrowing could compress your spinal nerve. But if you don't have any pain, why are you here?"

I was here because I was scared. I didn't know what was going on with my body. I didn't know if I could keep going. So I told him my story about my drifting left foot, how it sometimes felt like it was giving way. "But when I hiked the entire Camino using hiking poles, my gait was great. No limping, weakness, or left foot drift."

I decided to take the final plunge with full disclosure. "With this spinal stenosis diagnosis, is it still okay for me to hike the Grand Canyon with my daughter in October? I'll use my hiking poles. I just don't want to injure myself or make this worse."

Dr. Abode's head cocked. "You're going to hike the Grand Canyon?" He nodded. "Of course you are." He smiled. "Yes, it's okay for you to stick with your plans."

He turned serious again. "I'm going to run a few more tests on your muscles and nerves. Just want to make sure there's nothing else going on."

Then he paused, leaned forward, looked hard at me. "Sandi, you will eventually need surgery. But I will do everything I can to delay surgery as long as possible to allow you to continue what you're doing, to live this life that makes you so happy. For now, just keep walking and staying active."

Now I had two doctors telling me to stay the course. Medical advice I was delighted to follow. And I could still do the rim-to-rim! I did *not* want to carry one more incomplete goal over to next year. *Who knows what will happen in 2020?*

I chanted a new walking manta. *My spine will be fine. I'm staying active and have no pain. I can do this and be strong enough to finish my 75th birthday list.*

This was not the summer I had planned, but things were still working out. I started walking earlier in the morning to avoid the blistering heat. I climbed the stairs at the 100 Bridge and the lighthouse four to five times a week. I still had more than a month of training and was determined to make the best of it.

Jonathan and the boys came down for the weekend, as they had most of the summer. While the boys and Arnie played in the pool, Jonathan and I went out for our usual 5k along our favorite ICW path. We started chatting about our plans for walking the gnarly, swampy 13.6K Bulow Park Trail Run in December.

We walked in silence for a while. He had been such a solid, supportive walking partner, especially during this past summer with all its twists and turns. Jonathan loved to tease, but he knew full well how worried I was about the Grand Canyon. "Mom, you have done the hard work, walked every day even in this crazy heat, climbed the steps at the bridge and the lighthouse. You and Rachel will do fine. You two make a great team. You're both warriors. Enjoy this journey. I'm so proud of you."

He was beginning to sound like his dad.

It was September 2019, Friday the 13th. "I'm going to call the North Rim," I told Arnie after I finished lunch and headed to my office.

"I already checked the website this morning and nothing was open," said Arnie.

"Thanks, hon. I just feel the need to call."

I took a deep breath, called the number. This time a human answered. "Grand Canyon Forever North Rim reservations, how can I help you?"

"Hi, this is a long shot, but do you have any lodging open for Wednesday, October 2nd of *this* year?" I wasn't taking any chances with the wrong date!

She paused for a minute as she searched. "You called at just the right time. We received a few last-minute cancellations earlier today, and it looks like you may be in luck. In fact, we have two options for October 2nd, the Western or the Frontier. The Western is more expensive because it's right on the Rim. The Frontier is very nice too and it's $100 cheaper."

"Is the Western one of those cabins that has the front porch with rocking chairs looking out over the canyon?"

"Yes, it is. There are only six of these cabins on the Rim, and this is the best one. It has the biggest view and it's right by the Lodge."

I was gob smacked. "This is a dream come true! I've seen the pictures of this cabin on the website and it's beautiful. This may be my last visit to the North Rim. It's for my 75th year, and my daughter and I are going to be there just one night, but we would be staying in the best cabin on the North Rim!" I took a breath, stopped babbling.

She chuckled. "Reserve the Western. You won't be sorry."

I still couldn't believe it. "Are you *sure* you're for real? You're not a scam operation? You're not a robot? You are a Forever Representative, right?"

She laughed. "I'm for real."

I took the Western. And so for a few hours Thursday morning, October 3rd, we will sit in our rocking chairs on the front porch of the best cabin on the North Rim enjoying the Grand Canyon panorama.

Summer ended. It was time to leave. I got up three hours early, so Arnie and I had time to sit and chat with no time pressure. The driver arrived. I gathered my stuff. We kissed goodbye. "You and Rachel will be fine. Love you. Be careful. Keep me posted. Have fun."

Arnie had served as my life preserver and anchor through these turbulent summer storms.

I learned that boulders on a trail don't have to become impassable barriers. They just provide a reason to adjust, forge a new path. They can even bring out the best in myself and others and strengthen relationships.

The word *resilience* has taken on a more powerful meaning for me. This summer taught me that it's more than just bouncing back. Problems can either weaken your resolve or deepen your determination. Nobody said achieving big dreams would be easy. Find a way. Do it anyway. Enjoy the journey.

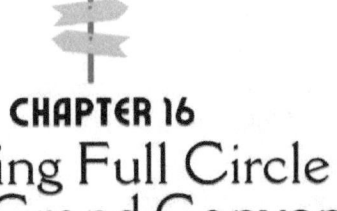

CHAPTER 16

Coming Full Circle at the Grand Canyon

"There's no question about it, the rim-to-rim hike in Grand Canyon National Park is a classic bucket list adventure. But it's no stroll in the park, that's for sure. Being unprepared can have catastrophic results. However, when you've trained properly, have the right gear, and know what to expect, it can be one of the most memorable experiences of your life. For the hearty souls who are willing to work for it—less than one percent of the Grand Canyon's five million annual visitors— the real magic lies below the rim."

—National Park Blog

Rachel and I were eating lunch at Maswik Lodge on the South Rim of the Grand Canyon. Stress had started seeping in. "Rachel, maybe we should we start earlier than 5:00 tomorrow morning. Maybe 3:30 or even 2:30? They're forecasting a temperature spike."

I paused. "Maybe we should even start at midnight tonight. What do you think?"

Rachel nodded, smiled. "That sounds like a great idea, Mom. We're comfortable hiking Bright Angel in the dark with our headlamps. Let's go get our backpacks ready. We're still tired from our travel so we can get some sleep before we head out."

It was Tuesday, only our second day of acclimating and recovering at the canyon. We were still sleep-deprived from Rachel's Ironman trip and jet-lagged from the flight from

Baltimore, but this was about as good as it would get given our short time frame.

Later, we were in bed. Eyes shut. Brain buzzing. No sleep. I rested for 30 minutes. Looked out the window at the sunny sky. *No way am I going to sleep, I'm too hyper. Maybe we should just head out now.* I looked over at Rachel. She wasn't moving, so I closed my eyes.

A moment later Rachel stirred. "Mom, are you awake? I can't sleep at all. I wonder if we should just head out now."

"Yes! I thought you were sleeping. Let's go. This way we'll get to hike almost all the way to Indian Garden before it's totally dark. We'll end up hiking all through the night, but if we can't sleep, we're going to be even more tired if we wait until midnight to start."

We packed up, walked to the Bright Angel trailhead and asked someone to take our picture just a few minutes after 5:00 p.m. The curving trail was familiar. The erosion-prevention rocks and mounds seemed a bit more precarious than I remembered. I clenched my hiking poles and gingerly stepped over each one, sometimes tensing up when my foot slipped slightly on the sandy trail. My eyes were glued on the trail, but I occasionally allowed myself to gaze up at the end-of-day lightshow in the sky and down at the plumb-colored shadows creeping across the craggy canyon basin below.

The yellow, orange, and red hues of the setting sun grew in intensity. But when the sun started to slip from view, and the canyon darkened, our initial adrenalin rush started to wane.

We still found little things to celebrate, such as getting to 3 Mile Resthouse before darkness completely descended. The trail smoothed out a bit from then on. It would be easier to walk on this section with headlamps.

"Okay, Mom, I'm sure I'm going to say this a few more times, but I'm so glad we left early. We've already hiked more than three miles in daylight, got to enjoy all the beautiful sunset views, and we have less than 21 miles left to the North Rim trailhead." Rachel laughed.

That sounds just like the pep talk I gave Rachel back in 1991. Sweet.

"I agree," I said. "It's much easier to be here in the dark on this trail. Jacob's Ladder is not as steep as the first 3 miles, and best of all, it's just a little more than 1.5 miles to Indian Garden."

We were totally alone. The last people we saw were at 1.5 Mile Resthouse. The sky grew darker. I stopped talking, and with that special mother-daughter radar, Rachel could tell I was getting tired and needed some pepping up. "Mom, isn't it somewhere along here where you gave your 'Don't stop now' speech to me, Rob, and the boys when we were here a few years ago in July?"

I laughed, immediately energized. "Oh, yes. It was July and hot. You all wanted to turn around and hike back out. We sat on a ledge in the shade somewhere right along here. I knew we were less than a mile from Indian Garden with leafy cottonwood trees, lots of shade, fresh drinking water, and even that little stream. I remember saying: 'We are so close to the cool! Please don't turn back now. For the rest of your life, you will be able to look down from the South Rim and see that white strip out to Plateau Point and know that you hiked that very trail. You will never, ever forget this hike.'"

Rachel stopped and turned. Even in the dark, I could tell she was smiling. "So, we did it," Rachel said. "The Plateau Trail was wide and flat, everything you said it would be. And even though it was hot, being able to look down at the olive-green Colorado River snaking through the bottom of the canyon was incredible. You gave us the gift of a spectacular milestone and memory."

My daughter typically doesn't talk much on long hikes and here she was trying to distract me the same way I did with her on our first hike all those years ago.

My spirits grew brighter as stars started twinkling in the velvet blue sky. We turned away from the rocky, rugged canyon wall, and followed the trail through tall cottonwoods into the familiar Indian Garden rest stop. We stopped at our favorite giant tree, a place of many fond memories and where I want some of my ashes scattered.

"Let's fill our bottles and go back to the restrooms to eat something. I'm getting cold," Rachel said.

"Good idea." We had less than 20 miles left.

We sat on the floor by the clean compostable toilet as we ate and drank. Thank goodness neither of us was having any trouble eating like Rachel did on that first hike when she was 15. We had traveled so far since then, getting stronger, smarter, more trail savvy.

We started off strong after leaving Indian Garden, but then I slipped off a rock in the middle of a stream.

I was jarred. My foot was drenched. I scolded myself. *You have got to be more careful!* I was scared. *I'm already starting to lose steam. This can't be happening so early in the hike. I know I'm stronger than this. The last thing I want to do is make Rachel worry. I can do this! Nobody said this would be easy. I have to dig deep and find my reservoir of strength!*

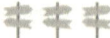

The trail widened. Garden Creek bubbled on our left. Then we entered Devil's Corkscrew hiking down at night in the cool. My emotions swayed back and forth as we zigzagged down and around the switchbacks. Back and forth, positive and negative. I was glad we left early but frustrated with my pace. I know how positive I can be. Always able to find a way to get it done. But I can't seem to shake this lurking, looming fear. Somehow, I have to find my trustworthy source of energy buried under this heavy blanket of fatigue.

Sandi! Get a grip! You are back on this beautiful trail, finally hiking it with Rachel after all those years of surgeries, injuries, and issues. You're slow, but you're doing fine. And remember, you'll hike much faster once we start hiking across the bottom. Now that's the spirit!

My inner pep talk lasted for a while as we eased off Corkscrew and balanced carefully on slippery rocks across a few streams. Thank goodness for my hiking poles! The next section was particularly daunting since it was where I slipped and tore a ligament when Carole and I had hiked down ten years ago.

I started a mantra. *Step carefully. Watch your step. These rocks are big and slimy. It's easy to slip and fall.* So far so good. I started again. *Step carefully Watch your step...* "Damn!" My foot slipped. I banged into a boulder.

"Mom! Are you okay?" Rachel turned around.

"I'm sorry I frightened you. I started to slip on a rock and just allowed myself to hit this boulder rather than twist my ankle. My hip is a little sore, but my foot is fine."

"But are you okay? You've been really quiet. That's not like you and I'm afraid you're getting discouraged. We're doing fine, Mom. You know that don't you? We're slow, but we're finally doing it together. Are you sure you're okay?"

"I am, hon. Thank you."

We hiked even more slowly over the rocky trail. Doing my best to stay upbeat and confident. Still struggling to force back my fatigue. And now I was making Rachel worry. The last thing I wanted to do!

Dig deeper. Find your strength. You know you can do this! We are going to do this! The sky grew pitch black, the stars more brilliant. Memories started twinkling in my brain. I smiled as I thought of her solo hike across the canyon and our gleeful reunion on the North Rim after I had shuttled over to meet her. I remembered all our shorter hikes in the canyon, even if it was just down to our favorite 3 Mile Resthouse. We have always found a way to enjoy the canyon. *But this year we are going all the way in one day. Finally, finally we are here hiking it together again after all these years!*

The trail turned and the sounds of the Colorado River swept up the canyon. Then, as if we needed any more reason to celebrate, we stepped onto the sandy portion of River Trail. No rocks. Just sand. Usually hiking on this sand is a royal pain, but not tonight. My head talk was faster than my feet. *We made it to the sand. Every little step brings us closer to the bridge. Just one more mile. Just one more mile.*

"Oh, Mom. I just saw something that will make you very happy."

Her headlamp reflected off Silver Bridge. The perfect shiny motivator!

I gasped, "What a beautiful sight!" We made it to the bottom of the canyon! This was a huge milestone! We walked across the suspension bridge slung over the Colorado River. We had hiked down almost 10 miles, descending at least 4,500 feet. It was 1:20 a.m. We had been hiking for more than 8 hours. Slow? Oh, yes. Fun and beautiful? That too. Most of the way.

We bypassed Bright Angel Campground, walked across a small bridge over Bright Angel Creek, and headed toward Phantom Ranch. Soon we saw lights and took the side trail through the beautiful settlement of hikers' cabins built out of wood and stone. *Phantom Ranch! Excited to reach this landmark filled with memories. It's been so many years.*

We walked by the canteen and came to a brand-new compostable bathroom structure with steps leading up to a covered porch with three doors. "Mom," Rachel said. "You wait here. I'm going to go to check this out."

I sat on a rock, my aching fatigue creeping back in. *I've hiked this trail through the night before on so many canyon crossings and felt fine. I never even yawned! I guess my age is finally catching up to me.*

Rachel came down the stairs. "Mom, we need to rest. There's nobody else on the trail. This place is clean and not even close to the campground. There's room for us to take our bags inside, eat, and maybe even sleep for an hour or so. What do you think?"

I nodded. Rachel grabbed my backpack and took my arm. We climbed up the steps, organized our backpacks on the hard, clean floor, and broke out our feast of chips and cookies. Around 3:00, we scrunched up on the floor on our space blankets with our backpacks as pillows and drifted off.

I woke about 20 minutes later to pee. I was curled up right by the toilet, but there was no way I could get up quietly or gracefully. I rolled over, planted my artificial knees beneath me, ignored the feeling of implants grinding on the hard floor, and gradually struggled to my feet. My space blanket rattled with every move, so I ended up waking Rachel. Twenty minutes later, it started all over again. And again. After two hours of resting and rattling, it was time to get moving.

We opened the door and were greeted by trickles of daylight that had managed to seep through the recesses of the dark canyon. Back at the canteen, we sat at the picnic table across from each other, eating snack cookies and drinking coffee. I gazed at Rachel and remembered our first hike as we sat in this same spot, maybe even this same table. Back then she was sobbing. *What have I done?* I remember asking myself. *Is this too much? Will this be our last big adventure? Will she be too discouraged because we didn't do the entire hike?* Seeing her so depleted and discouraged was scary. That's when the *trail angel* stepped up with her protein powder. It had been my first encounter with these seemingly celestial beings. And these creatures had continued to emerge through the years just when they were needed the most.

We made it back then. And with this little rest and new burst of energy, I knew we would make it now.

Our spirits lifted and the sky brightened as we left Phantom Ranch around 6:00 a.m. "Rachel," I said, "we've already hiked more than 10 miles, which means we have fewer than 14 miles left to the North Rim trailhead, just a little longer than a half marathon. Then just another 1.7 miles to the lodge. And these next 7 miles across the bottom of the canyon to Cottonwood are easy and beautiful." I was trying to pump us both up.

Soon we entered the deep inner gorge sliced in the middle by Bright Angel Creek. "Hon, do you remember anything about this section of the trail?

"Is this the box?"

"Right! The dreaded box that Sid Hirsh told us to avoid crossing when the sun is directly overhead since it can turn into an oven. We crossed through early last time we hiked together and we're crossing through even earlier today!"

We emerged from the box before 8:00. It was still shady with no direct sun overhead. "We have a little more than three miles to Cottonwood," I said, delighted with our progress.

The wide expanse of the inner canyon was spectacular. We stopped for a few pictures. Then moved forward with Rachel walking ahead on the undulating trail across the magical middle canyon. My footsteps hit the dirt with a Whomp! Whomp! Whomp! That sound slowly morphed into a nagging Why? Why? Why?

Why is this so important? Why do you have to do it in one day? Why don't you be reasonable? Take the time to smell the roses? Take it easy and just do a shorter hike? Or camp along the way? Why did you have to do it this year when it was so hard to fit everything in? Why do you put yourself through this? And your daughter?

Because. Because. Because.

Because I want to. I need to. I have taken my time and thoroughly enjoyed the canyon on many other shorter hikes. Because the one-day rim-to-rim has been embedded in my soul for so long. It's a part of me. And Rachel and I never had the opportunity to complete the entire R2R and hike up the North Rim together. Because we have been waiting 28 years to finish what we started.

I took a deep breath. *Because I might be getting too old to do this hike and I'm scared to let it go. I love being in my 70s. I just don't want to get so old that I can't do this. I can't let it go. I'm not ready to let it go. Not yet. Not now.*

We kept walking, surrounded by sage brush, boulders, and even flowers as we hiked along the trail under the giant dome of crisp azure sky. Rachel and I were the only two people in the whole world walking right through the heart of this sacred space.

We were hiking our rim-to-rim. Together. All the way. In one day.

Another hiker came running from behind, around us, ahead, then skidded to a stop. "Good morning! How are you doing? Nice to finally see someone else on the trail." We could tell he was in a big hurry, so we answered quickly and wished him well as he turned to continue his run.

"We should start seeing the cottonwood trees any moment now," I said. "I'm pretty sure the campground is just around this corner. Oh yes, there it is!"

"Look, Mom," Rachel said as she bent down and picked up a multi-colored laminated chart in the middle of the trail with mileage, milestones, and time estimates for a rim-to-rim-to-rim. "I saw this dangling from that runner's backpack. He is going to be devastated when he sees he's lost it. I could just leave it on the trail and hope he finds it, but I bet we'll see him on his way back. I'll keep it and we can watch for him."

"Good idea," I agreed. "Here we are. Shall we stop at this picnic bench and eat something?"

"It's 10:00 o'clock, so it took us around four hours to hike the 7.6 miles from Phantom," I said as I watched Rachel happily surveying our array of snacks on the picnic table. My thoughts again flew back 28 years when we sat in this area and I was trying to get her to eat something, anything before we started up the steep North Rim trail.

Now all these years later, Rachel was worried about my 75-

year-old somewhat finicky stomach. She was delighted to see me eat. We both appreciated our changing roles.

It was around 10:45 as we stepped onto the wide trail with just 1.4 miles from Cottonwood to the Manzanita Rest Area. *This section shouldn't take too long*, I thought. But that thought was abruptly adjusted. Although the incline was gentle, the blazing sun was not. By the time we got to Manzanita, I was feeling dizzy, trying to ignore the feeling, wish it away. "Mom, are you okay?" asked my eagle-eyed daughter.

"Um, I know we just filled up with water at Cottonwood, but I think I need to sit for a bit and drink. Then I'll be fine."

"Mom, after this you need to tell me if you're not feeling well so we can stop right then. You can't pretend. I need to trust you to be honest with me and not wait until I ask you," Rachel scolded.

"You're right. I'm sorry. I'll be upfront and honest from now on." When I went over to fill my water bottle, I could hear Rachel rearranging her backpack. Then I saw out of the corner of my eye that she was rummaging through mine, taking things out and putting them in hers to lighten my load. She was worried. I did not need to add to her stress.

When we got back on the trail, the runner came bounding back down toward us. Rachel waved the milestone card. "I think we found something of yours."

"Oh, yes! My time and milestone graph keeps me focused and motivated. I felt lost without it. Thank you so much!"

"You're welcome," said Rachel. "Have a great run."

"And you two have a great hike. Thanks again!"

It was past noon with full sun and getting hotter as we continued our North Rim climb. I remembered this 3-mile section up to Redwall Bridge from previous hikes many years ago as being relatively easy, especially compared to the switchbacks after the bridge. But my pace had slowed to a crawl and my thinking started getting hazy. My body could not overcome the lack of sleep. My adrenaline was sapped. My shoes gained weight.

Like I was hiking through Jell-O.

This was not at all how I had pictured this hike. I knew it would be hard. That I'd have to rely on mind over matter. But my "matter" was not cooperating.

We reached the Roaring Springs turnoff. My fog cleared briefly as we looked down the little spur trail. "Mom, when I did that rim to rim alone a few years ago, I carried that 3x5 milestone card you made for me, and I would have been devastated if I had lost it. It was my trail guide and inspiration since you had included estimated times at each milestone."

Rachel's comments touched my heart. She remembered! "I love those little 3x5 cards I made for every hike," I said. "When I'm cleaning out a drawer or looking through a photo album, I still find them. I never threw any away, but I forgot to put dates on most of them, so I can't remember what year it was. Crazy."

"How are you feeling, Mom?

I responded honestly. "I feel fine, not dizzy at all, just hazy, exhausted, although this little stop helped clear my mind. If I remember correctly, this is one of the prettiest sections of the hike with waterfalls and brilliant rock formations."

"When was the last time you hiked up the North Rim?" Rachel asked, trying to pep me up. She knew how much I love telling Grand Canyon stories.

"Let me think. It was in May 1998, so 21 years ago. That was my last rim-to-rim-to-rim. I was 54. Later on after we moved, I'd occasionally fly back to Tucson. Carole and I would come up and hike. We hiked all the way to Cottonwood two times, more than 30 miles. I kept dreaming at some point I could do a few more rim-to-rim-to-rims, but it never happened."

We slipped back into our own thoughts. My pace slowed even more, the haze returned, but my legs kept moving. Finally, we reached Redwall Bridge. It was 3:15 p.m. Almost four hours since we left Cottonwood. More than one hour a mile.

It was here on the first switchback right after the bridge that

Rachel and I had met up with Sid Hirsh and made the decision to turn around. That was 28 years ago. But today there was no turning back. The next milestone was Supai Tunnel. How hard could it be? It was only six-tenths of a mile.

Well darn, I thought as we rounded our second switchback. *I expected the switchbacks, but I sure don't remember these big logs. I'll bet they put these on the trail after it washed out a few years ago.*

I started needing Rachel's help lifting my legs over some of the higher logs. She would step back, take the pole from my right hand so I could rest it on her shoulder, then I would lean on her and brace the pole in my left hand to climb over the log without tripping. It was quite a process.

Just before we got to Supai Tunnel, we saw two young men bouncing down the trail. "Hi! Hey! Mother and daughter? How cool. Where did you guys come from?"

"We started at the South Rim almost 24 hours ago around 5:00 p.m.," said Rachel.

"The South Rim? No kidding!" Their smiles grew even bigger.

"But we did have to sleep in the restroom at Phantom Ranch for a few hours," I added.

They laughed. "Even better! What a great story. And you're almost to the top. It must be fabulous hiking the whole thing without carrying heavy backpacks."

"It's the best. Where are you headed?" Rachel asked since it seemed like a strange time to be starting a hike down the North Rim without a backpack.

"Oh, we camped at Cottonwood last night and hiked out this morning. We're staying at the Lodge. But our friend wanted to spend some time at Roaring Springs and we haven't heard from him, so we're going down to check. He probably just lost track of time. We better get going. Congratulations, you two!" They called as they headed down, easily flying around the switchbacks and sailing over the logs.

Their enthusiasm was briefly contagious as we hiked through the soft shade of Supai Tunnel. It's funny how some people can spread joy without even being aware of their impact. Those two happy hikers earned the title of *trail angels*.

We enter the tree-lined section of the trail. These North Rim miles after the tunnel are surely the longest I have ever hiked. My spirits lift, but cement still seems to gather and gain weight on the soles of my shoes. I just need to get to Coconino Overlook. Then I know I can make it. But I am so slow! My legs so heavy.

"There's a flat rock, hon. I need to sit." And so, I sit. Then we step slowly forward. Rachel hiking ahead, doing her best to set the pace. Showing me the way. I move from rock to rock. I see a flat spot. I sit. Rachel steps back. Shares her water bottle. I sip. I survey the bountiful array of goodies Rachel has removed from her heavy pack and scattered across my lap. *Fritos!* I snack. I smile at Rachel. I squint, strive to remember this section of the trail. She holds out her hand, helping me to stand. I move forward, ten, twenty, thirty steps.

At 5:30, the first stage of sunset, we arrive at Coconino Overlook. We pause and savor the glistening panorama from the bird's eye balcony of this iconic Grand Canyon vista. Each rock strata brilliantly reflects its own color in the setting sun.

It slowly registered that we had been on the trail for more than 24 hours. We had been out of contact with our family since we started our hike yesterday. Of course, this was another thing on Rachel's mind as she kept checking for service on her phone while coaxing me up the trail. She knew Andrew and Rob would be frantic and hoped they had called Arnie, who would reassure them.

We turned away from the Overlook and headed up the final

.7 mile to the trailhead. Then Rachel glanced at her phone. "Wonderful! We've got service. Mom, go ahead up the trail. I'm going to text everyone and let them know we're okay."

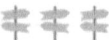

We arrived at the North Rim trailhead at around 6:00 p.m., hiking almost twenty-four miles in just over twenty-five hours. Could even be a record for the slowest "one-day" rim-to-rim. Didn't matter right now. We were finally together at the North Rim!

"It's less than two miles to the Lodge. How hard can that be?" I said, trusting that my usual end-of-hike adrenaline rush would finally kick in and carry me forward. But my anticipated euphoria refused to emerge. We walked a little farther. I was disoriented by lights on the side of the trail and started fretting that we had missed a turn, gotten lost. I sat on a rock. For the first time since our hike started, I wondered if I could make it. Being slow was one thing. Being totally depleted was another. I was scared. So was Rachel.

Then, we heard familiar bouncing sounds coming up behind us. "Hi, Mother and Daughter. You made it. Congratulations!" It was them. The *trail angels* we met on the trail who had been on their way down to find their friend.

"Hi! We are really glad to see you. Did you find your friend? Is he okay?" Rachel asked.

"He's fine, but pretty sore. He twisted his ankle. We're heading back to the Lodge to get our car so we can drive back to the trailhead and pick him up."

"We were getting worried this is not the right trail. Are we heading in the right direction?" asked Rachel.

"Oh yes! The Lodge is straight ahead. You have about a mile to go. Good job!"

"Thank you!" We both called as they charged down the trail. Again, they had no idea what their quick stop meant. Their infectious enthusiasm and jubilant encouragement gave me the final boost I needed to get up and start moving.

About 15 minutes later, we saw lights ahead. "See, Mom," Rachel was talking in a slow coaxing voice. "We're walking by the motel rooms, and there are the cabins, just a few more steps.

Rachel's sweet voice came floating through my fog. It finally registered. "We are almost there! I can do this!" I started counting my steps, always my go-to approach for moving forward when I feel like I can't take another step. 10, 50, 100. I hit 150 steps, looked up and saw the Lodge! We made it! "Rachel, we did it! We completed our rim-to-rim! Together! We are here and we are fine!" She turned and looked at me with a triumphant smile as we faced and then embraced each other in the well-lit traffic circle in front of the Lodge. The morning of our first hike flashes through my mind and I remember the deer standing in the aura of that streetlight.

Still in charge, Rachel continued, "I think the pizza shop is closing. Let's go in quick to see if we can still buy something to eat. We need more than these trail snacks for dinner."

I stood bracing myself on the ice cream freezer, feeling dazed, watching Rachel talk earnestly with the young man at the cash register. "Mom, do you have some cash in your fanny pack? I convinced him to sell us his leftover pieces of pizza, but he can only take cash. And do you have enough for a tip? He is being so helpful."

I moved in slow motion as my fumbling fingers dug into the little pack around my waist where I kept my phone, medicine, and a few large bills. "Here, take it all. Give him a big tip. And please ask him for some salt packets."

She walked back to me with a big pizza box and a bigger smile. "We got their final few pieces. That was great timing!"

We walked back into the chilly night and into the lodge. Rachel went to the Tour Desk to grab our overnight bags. I gazed into the dining room, saw the clock by the reservation desk, and laughed. It was 7:50. We had made it in time for our 8:00 dinner reservations! Of course, there was no way we'd go. But it was a nice thought.

We checked in. The desk clerk saw the fatigue etched in our faces. "You are in luck. Your cabin is the closest one on the North Rim. All you do is walk down the steps through the back door of the lobby, go across the patio and up to the steps of your cabin. Good planning!" He gave us our keys and an encouraging smile.

The room was beautiful, with two queen-sized beds, even a gas fireplace. It was rustic and roomy. After my shower, I crawled into bed and sat with my back propped on the pillows. Rachel pulled up a little table with a few pieces of pizza and a cup of hot tea. "Okay, Mom, please eat and drink. I'm going to take my shower."

I took a bite and a sip, then slipped down in my bed, telling myself, *I need to close my eyes for just a minute.*

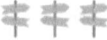

And then there was light. Morning. The cabin door was open.

"Mom, come out here, you've got to see this!" I crawled out of bed. Started for the door. Then stopped. The chill of mountain morning air blew in accompanied with soft hues of daylight.

I paused. I had to convince myself that we really had finished our hike up the North Rim, together, 28 years after our first attempt.

"Mom, hurry, you're going to miss it."

I walked out onto the porch and saw Rachel looking out at the brilliant sunrise, splashing glorious colors across that beautiful Grand Canyon. She turned to me and smiled. "We did it."

"We did." My eyes burned. Chest tightened. Tears flowed, matching the tears on her cheeks. We couldn't move. We just stood there looking at each other and the canyon light show, trying to catch our breath.

"I just want to point out," I laughed, as I sniffled and shivered, "I never once cried on the trail and you didn't either. You kept us moving, fueled, hydrated. You helped me step up and over those high steps and logs. I was in a fog. I don't remember some parts of the trail or the canyon, but I remember you."

"We did great," said Rachel as she wiped her tears. "Let's get ready and go get some breakfast. I'm hungry and you need to get some food in your stomach."

When I went into our cabin, I noticed Rachel had cleaned all the mud off my shoes. She had completely taken over as the mom of this mother-daughter team.

We walked gingerly into the cavernous dining room and checked out the breakfast buffet. Rachel was ravenous and dug right in, but suddenly my appetite vanished. I sat still, stared down at my plate, shook my head. "Rachel, I've always *loved* that feeling of leaving it all on the trail, knowing that I gave it every ounce of energy that was in me." I paused, catching my breath, grimacing. "But when I thought we might be lost on that final path to the lodge, it was the first time I ever felt like my well was totally dry, that I was running on empty. Almost every other big hike has ended with a bit of trail magic that lifted me up and helped me float to the end. That didn't happen this time."

"Mom, I've seen you tired before, but never as tired as you were last night. It was a scary moment for both of us. But after our hiker buddies reassured us, you got up and kept going the whole last mile without stopping. Maybe that's when the trail magic happened and you were just too tired to notice it."

Rachel paused between bites. "Usually at this point you're laughing and listing all the reasons we should be celebrating. I'm worried that you somehow view this as a failure just because it took so long and you got so tired. You did it, Mom. We did it. After all these years, we captured our dream. We aren't injured. Of course we're sore, but we earned every bit of that muscle pain. And we have great stories to tell, especially about sleeping in the

Phantom Ranch bathroom."

"You're right. We did it. I'm relieved. And happy. And thankful. You were wonderful, took such good care of me. It's just," I struggled, "I feel guilty, because even with everything to celebrate, it wasn't the ending I wanted."

I tried to perk up and eat, but finally pushed my plate away. "There's so much of the hike after Manzanita Rest Stop that I can't remember. This might be my last hike and I can't even picture the beauty of those glorious miles from Redwall Bridge to the top, those miles we finally got to hike together after all these years. It's like they didn't happen."

"Mom, you're still exhausted. Just give your brain a chance to catch up. I'll bet the memories will start coming back." Rachel shook her head, then burst out laughing. "Oh, my goodness, that sounds like something you would say. I'm turning into you!"

We both laughed. I pulled back my plate for a few more bites. After breakfast, we headed back to our cabin.

It was a joyful, never-ending morning. We returned to our porch, plunked down on our rocking chairs, read for a while, glanced up to enjoy the canyon, read a little more. Just what I had dreamed we'd do.

After lunch, we checked out, then walked out to the sunny patio of the North Rim Lodge. It was filled with Adirondack chairs, one of our favorite spots to sit, facing the rim, reading with our feet propped upon the low stone wall. Dozens of people were doing that very same thing today. "It's interesting, so many people are here when we saw so few on the trail," I said.

"Well, keep in mind there are lots of other day trips and hikes *normal* people take when they visit here. Not everybody does a rim-to-rim," Rachel laughed. She walked over to a group of women and asked if one of them could take our picture. They all smiled, and one jumped up right away. "Sure. Love to! So, you hiked over from the South Rim? That's great. When did you start?"

"We started Tuesday evening at 5:00, rested for a few hours at the bottom, and then hiked out last night. It took us 25 hours to get to the North Rim trailhead," I said, straight forward, no apology, no discounts, smiling at Rachel.

"That's amazing! I love that you did it as a mother and daughter team. When did you two start hiking together?"

We wanted to get going and didn't want to take too much of her time, but she kept peppering us with questions as we explained our journey from our first Grand Canyon hike in 1991 to this one.

Finally, we were able to slip in a few questions of our own and learned she and three other friends were heading out to do a North-South rim-to-rim early tomorrow morning. "We heard it's much easier going down the North Rim and up the South Rim. What do you think?"

"I think that's right," answered Rachel. "The South Rim is a thousand feet lower in elevation. It will still be a challenge at the end, especially the last three miles, but easier than the North Rim. Best wishes. Have a great hike."

We started to walk away. She called out to me. "Thank you for giving me the perfect picture of what I want to be when I'm 75. You are my inspiration. I'm heading out for my first trans-canyon hike around the same age you were when you did your first one!"

I was flattered, a little embarrassed. "Thank you! I wish you the best—for this hike and beyond."

We took the shuttle back to the South Rim, dropped our things off in our room and walked into the Maswik lobby to meet Carole, who had driven up from the strawbale house she and Mike had built down the road from the canyon. "Hi, you two!! It is so good to see you. You look great! I can't wait to hear how it went."

We hugged hard and went straight into the cafeteria, quickly getting our food so we could sit down and catch up. We shared our stories. "But you two seemed to do fine, right?" Carole said. "Just slow? No big deal. And no big surprise given how depleted you were when you started out. And Rachel, I can't believe you completed an Ironman just a few days before!"

"It's not what we planned, but we made it work. Mom was really tired, but I never felt like we were in danger because we were so well supplied."

"So, when do you head out?" Carole said.

"Tomorrow morning. On the way out we're going to stop at the Smokey Bear statue for some joint birthday pictures, since it's his 75th birthday this year too."

The next morning, I wrote a postcard for Rachel. "My dear daughter. You were the icing on the cake. Actually, you were the whole cake, the candles and even the plate! I love you so much, Mom." I knew she would love getting this surprise in the mail.

And Rachel had one final surprise for me when we stopped by Smokey Bear. She opened a bag and handed me an adorable plastic tiara just like the multi-color tiara I had received for my third-place Tri-for-a-Cure finish. Only this one boasted the number 75 on its crest. She also presented me with a "75 year" banner. The perfect attire for my birthday pictures with Smokey!

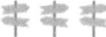

"We never gave up, Mom," said Rachel as we got back into the car. "All those years when it didn't work out. We held on, kept trying, always made the best of it. And every hike has always been fun and memorable. It's been part of our lives for so long, in such a good way."

I was still frustrated I couldn't remember everything on the final portion of the hike, especially after reaching Redwall Bridge. So, I made a resolution. *My picture isn't complete. It feels like too many pieces are still missing. I may have to accept that this is a puzzle that will never have all its pieces—but maybe not.*

Rachel could help me fill in those empty blanks in our story. She could remind me to celebrate that we finally did it. That it's already a beautiful picture. I keep thinking that maybe someday we can even return to fill in the missing pieces.

I know for sure this story is not over, not yet.

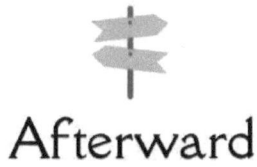

Afterward

Arnie was with me every step of the way as I wrote this book. He got it. He got me. He understood what a big deal this was for me to finally get my story out of my head onto paper and into print. He shared my joy. He sustained me every step of the way.

But we could not cross the finish line together.

Shortly after I finished my manuscript, Arnie died, unexpectedly, in the hospital.

My heart was broken. My soul shattered. At first it was impossible to move forward with anything—especially this book. But I knew Arnie would have none of that. He whispered. He pestered. He insisted. *I appreciate that you miss me, hon. But don't you dare use my death as an excuse to stop living your life, to stop doing all you love. You will honor me by moving forward. I know that and so do you. Get going.* And so I did.

The love of my family, especially Rachel and Jonathan, and the memories of my and Arnie's 54 years together helped me start moving again.

As I reviewed my manuscript one more time before submitting it to my publisher, I realized this book is a love letter to Arnie—his support, his encouragement, his faith in me. He made this life possible. I miss him so much. I wish he were here with me to celebrate. He would be so proud. And he would tell me, "I knew you could do it, hon. Never had any doubt."

Acknowledgments
Giving Thanks

Back in 2018, during our year-long celebration of our 50th anniversary, Arnie and I walked into breakfast at the Hilton Head Health Institute. He noticed a woman sitting alone. "Why don't you come eat with us?" You, Lynya Floyd, joined us.

Later, when you told us you were writing an article for a national magazine, I took the plunge and asked if you could help me get started writing my book. You said, "Start writing every day. Don't look through your journals. Don't do any research. Just write. Every day. You can always revise later." I listened. I wrote. Every day.

Without you, I'd still be digging through old journals. Researching instead of writing. You helped me get started, then served as my coach as I organized the fragments of my tale into an outline, and finally chapters. And then you gave me the biggest gift of all. You helped me believe in myself and my story so I could move forward on this long journey with confidence and joy. Thank you!

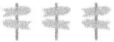

Thank you to my dear family and friends, members of my tribe.

At the starting line were Sandy West and Jane Ramsey, mentors who got me off on the right foot at Limited Brands and assured me I was on the right path when they read my introduction.

Sandy Hall, Susan Marshall, Donna Larsen, Suzanne Day, Nancy Brown, Deb Tinajero, and Jackie Witte also read, reviewed, and cheered me on as I headed out on my writing journey.

Patty Hartsfield, Ann Galloway, Cathy Kasriel, Jane Altenhofen, Wil Hessert, Art Dycke, Sherry McClain, Fred Ebrahimi, Kim Porter, Ileine Hoffman, Cheryle Easton, Maddy Kahn, Nancy Sasser, Anita Olson, Cindy Benz, and Cheryl Stippler joined in reading and pacing me along the way.

My entire Grand Haven book club, Page Turners, led by Peg Pettingell, listened to my updates, asked me questions, and celebrated every step forward and backward, the entire five years it took for me to write, revise, and edit this book.

Eight dear souls volunteered to go the distance and read the entire manuscript: Kathie Gargiulo, who asked lots of questions because she didn't know me well, and Carole Sheehan who offered helpful insights because she did. Two others in the book also asked to read it all. Ann Fazzini, the young woman I met in the van who insisted I could hike the Inca Trail. Mike Darzi, who provided even more encouragement with this book than he did during our years of One Day Hike adventures. Then Joan Klopf and Pat Malak helped me cross the finish line by volunteering to read the entire draft. Joan provided painstaking editing and proofing, thoughtful questions and challenges, and some tough love. Pat offered insightful feedback and much-needed encouragement by reacting passionately to the book and articulating how, who, and why my story would resonate with others. So did Lisa Herrington. And Melissa Bowersock, for also providing detailed feedback on the quality and emotional impact of my story.

Lynn Murphy, author and lifelong friend, provided feedback and assurance that that I had written a story worthy of sharing with others. She also introduced me to Thea Rademacher of Flint Hills

Publishing, a family-owned business. And that has made all the difference. Thea is my passionate, successful, caring publisher who assigned her son, Paul Fredrickson, to serve as my talented and capable editor. Thank you, Thea, for embracing me and my manuscript. Thank you, Paul, for seeing themes I could not see myself, urging me to dig deeper. Thank you for making this story flight-worthy, ready to send out into the world.

My family read portions and patiently listened to my updates, fears, insights, and worries, usually as we walked together. Assuring me. Encouraging me.

Thank you, grandsons Jonathan and Andrew Litz, Jonathan (Flip) and Samuel Richmond. Thank you, in-laws Rob Litz and Lauren Cortese, for your partnership and support.

Thank you, Jonathan, for our years and miles of walks and talks. For propping me up, offering your arm, your shoulder, your ear.

Thank you, Rachel, for sharing our Grand Canyon passion and sustaining us through the years as we kept moving forward, hiking canyons and mountains, switching caretaker roles, clinging to our dream.

And to my soulmate Arnie, who never failed to lift me up when I faltered, pull me together when I fell apart, anchor me when I started to drift, and through it all, make me laugh. I could not have made this journey without you by my side. Love you. Thank you. Love you even more.

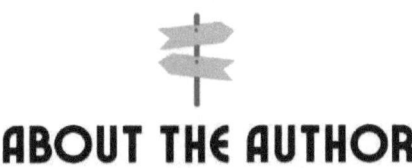

ABOUT THE AUTHOR

Sandra Richmond, PhD, did not fully embrace her active lifestyle until her mid-40s. Despite having arthritis, atrial fibrillation, spinal stenosis, and joint replacement surgeries in both hips and knees, she has slow-walked several marathons, half marathons, 50, 15, 10, and 5Ks, supporting worthy causes and happily encouraging others to join her in these walker-friendly events. She has completed events with every member of her family, creating unique and precious memories. After 70, Sandra incorporated adventure travel into her post-retirement life and has taken on challenging treks including the Inca Trail in Peru and the Camino de Santiago in Spain. She divides her time between Maryland and Florida.

Milepost 75 is her first book. She recently turned 80 and plans to celebrate this exciting new milepost all year long.

www.milepoststories.com

www.ingramcontent.com/pod-product-compliance
Lightning Source LLC
Chambersburg PA
CBHW021715120626
46545CB00004B/1573